T0401508

GOVERNMENT REPORTS ON HEALTH CARE FOR MARCH 2019

HEALTH CARE IN TRANSITION

Additional books and e-books in this series can be found
on Nova's website under the Series tab.

GOVERNMENT REPORTS ON HEALTH CARE FOR MARCH 2019

ERIC BEYER
EDITOR

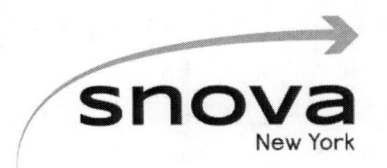

NOTICE TO THE READER

Library of Congress Cataloging-in-Publication Data

ISBN: 978-1-53615-844-1

Published by Nova Science Publishers, Inc. † New York

CONTENTS

Preface   **vii**

Chapter 1   Air Ambulance: Available Data Show Privately-
Insured Patients Are at Financial Risk   **1**
United States Government Accountability Office

Chapter 2   Defense Health Care:
DOD's Proposed Plan for Oversight of
Graduate Medical Education Programs   **29**
United States Government Accountability Office

Chapter 3   Drug Policy: Preliminary Observations
on the 2019 National Drug Control Strategy   **47**
Triana McNeil and Mary Denigan-Macauley

Chapter 4   Medicare and Medicaid:
CMS Should Assess Documentation
Necessary to Identify Improper Payments   **63**
United States Government Accountability Office

Chapter 5   Private Health Insurance:
Enrollment Remains Concentrated among
Few Issuers, Including in Exchanges   **123**
United States Government Accountability Office

Index **215**

Related Nova Publications **221**

PREFACE

This book is a comprehensive compilation of all reports, testimony, correspondence and other publications issued by the GAO (Government Accountability Office) during the month of March, grouped according to the topic: Health Care.

Chapter 1 - Air ambulances provide emergency services for critically ill patients. Relatively few patients receive such transports, but those who do typically have no control over the selection of the provider, which means privately-insured patients may be transported by out-of-network providers. The Joint Explanatory Statement accompanying the 2017 Consolidated Appropriations Act includes a provision for GAO to review air ambulance services. Among other objectives, this chapter describes (1) the extent of out-ofnetwork transports and balance billing and (2) the approaches selected states have taken to limit potential balance billing. GAO analyzed a private health insurance data set for air ambulance transports with information on network status and prices charged in 2017 (the most recent data available). Although this was the most complete data identified, the data may not be representative of all private insurers. In addition, GAO interviewed officials in six states (Florida, Maryland, Montana, New Mexico, North Dakota, and Texas) selected in part for variation in approaches to limit balance billing and location. GAO also interviewed air ambulance providers, health insurers, and Centers for

Medicare & Medicaid Services and Department of Transportation (DOT) officials. DOT provided technical comments on a draft of this chapter, which GAO incorporated as appropriate, and the Department of Health and Human Services had no comments.

Chapter 2 - DOD's health care system prepares medical personnel for wartime or humanitarian missions while providing health care to servicemembers and other eligible beneficiaries. It is responsible for ensuring that military servicemembers are physically and mentally fit to perform their missions and that it has an adequate number of medical personnel with the requisite skills and training to meet DOD's mission needs (operational medical force readiness). DOD uses GME programs to recruit and retain military physicians by providing specialized medical training through physician residencies and fellowships in exchange for active duty service obligations. The NDAA 2017 included a provision for GAO to review DOD's GME oversight process, as detailed in DOD's July 2018 report to Congress. GAO assessed to what extent DOD's proposed oversight process, as outlined in its report to Congress, addressed each of the NDAA 2017 requirements. GAO compared DOD's process with the NDAA 2017 requirements; reviewed relevant documentation, such as minutes from planning meetings and charters for two new oversight entities; and interviewed DOD officials. In commenting on a draft of this chapter, DOD did not fully agree with GAO's finding that the department had not developed plans to implement its new GME oversight process, citing as a basis certain preliminary steps it had taken. Based on the preliminary nature of these steps and other reasons explained in the report, GAO stands by its finding.

Chapter 3 - Over 70,000 people died from drug overdoses in 2017, according to the most recently available Centers for Disease Control and Prevention data. Overdoses have become the leading cause of death due to injuries in the United States, and most of these deaths involve opioids. GAO has a body of work on drug policy and ongoing work on ONDCP's efforts, including issuance of the National Drug Control Strategy. GAO also noted in its March 2019 High Risk report that federal efforts to prevent drug misuse is an emerging issue requiring close attention. This statement includes preliminary GAO observations on the 2019 National Drug Control Strategy and related findings from select GAO reports on federal opioid-related efforts. It is based on ongoing GAO work, two reports that GAO issued in March 2018 and October 2017, and selected updates on recommendations from these reports as of February 2019. For ongoing work and recommendation updates, GAO assessed the 2019 National Drug Control Strategy against statutory requirements, reviewed ONDCP and HHS documents, and interviewed ONDCP officials.

Chapter 4 - In fiscal year 2017, Medicare FFS had an estimated $23.2 billion in improper payments due to insufficient documentation, while Medicaid FFS had $4.3 billion—accounting for most of the programs' estimated FFS medical review improper payments. Medicare FFS coverage policies are generally national, and the program directly pays providers, while Medicaid provides states flexibility to design coverage policies, and the federal government and states share in program financing. Among other things, GAO examined: (1) Medicare and Medicaid documentation requirements and factors that contribute to improper payments due to insufficient documentation; and (2) the extent to which Medicaid reviews provide states with actionable information. GAO reviewed Medicare and Medicaid documentation requirements and improper payment data for fiscal years 2005 through 2017, and interviewed officials from CMS, CMS contractors, and six state Medicaid programs. GAO selected the states based on, among other criteria, variation in estimated state improper payment rates, and FFS spending and enrollment.

Chapter 5 - A highly concentrated health insurance market may indicate less competition and could affect consumers' choice of issuers and the premiums they pay. In 2014, PPACA required the establishment of health insurance exchanges—a new type of marketplace where individuals and small groups can compare and select among insurance plans sold by participating issuers—and the introduction of other reforms that could affect market concentration and competition among issuers. GAO previously reported that enrollment through these newly established exchanges was also generally concentrated. PPACA included a provision for GAO to study market concentration. This chapter describes changes in the concentration of enrollment among issuers in (1) overall individual, small group, and large group markets, and (2) individual and small group exchanges. GAO determined market share in the overall markets using enrollment data from 2015 and 2016 that issuers are required to report annually to the Centers for Medicare & Medicaid Services (CMS) and compared that data to 2011 through 2014 enrollment data GAO analyzed in previous reports. GAO determined market share in the exchanges from 2015 through 2017 using other sources of enrollment data from CMS and states. For all data sets, GAO used the most recent data available.

In: Government Reports on Health Care ...   ISBN: 978-1-53615-844-1
Editor: Eric Beyer   © 2019 Nova Science Publishers, Inc.

Chapter 1

AIR AMBULANCE: AVAILABLE DATA SHOW PRIVATELY-INSURED PATIENTS ARE AT FINANCIAL RISK*

United States Government Accountability Office

ABBREVIATIONS

ADA	Airline Deregulation Act of 1978
ADAMS	Atlas & Database of Air Medical Services
DOT	U.S. Department of Transportation
ERISA	Employee Retirement Income Security Act of 1974
FAA	Federal Aviation Administration

---

* This is an edited, reformatted and augmented version of the United States Government Accountability Office Report to the Chairwoman, Committee on Education and the Workforce, House of Representatives, Publication No. GAO-19-292, dated March 2019.

WHY GAO DID THIS STUDY

Air ambulances provide emergency services for critically ill patients. Relatively few patients receive such transports, but those who do typically have no control over the selection of the provider, which means privately-insured patients may be transported by out-of-network providers.

The Joint Explanatory Statement accompanying the 2017 Consolidated Appropriations Act includes a provision for GAO to review air ambulance services. Among other objectives, this chapter describes (1) the extent of out-ofnetwork transports and balance billing and (2) the approaches selected states have taken to limit potential balance billing.

GAO analyzed a private health insurance data set for air ambulance transports with information on network status and prices charged in 2017 (the most recent data available). Although this was the most complete data identified, the data may not be representative of all private insurers. In addition, GAO interviewed officials in six states (Florida, Maryland, Montana, New Mexico, North Dakota, and Texas) selected in part for variation in approaches to limit balance billing and location. GAO also interviewed air ambulance providers, health insurers, and Centers for Medicare & Medicaid Services and Department of Transportation (DOT) officials. DOT provided technical comments on a draft of this chapter, which GAO incorporated as appropriate, and the Department of Health and Human Services had no comments.

WHAT GAO FOUND

Privately-insured patients transported by air ambulance providers outside of their insurers' provider networks are at financial risk for balance bills—which, as the figure shows, are for the difference between prices charged by providers and payments by insurers. Any balance bills are in addition to copayments or other types of cost-sharing typically paid by patients under their insurance coverage.

According to GAO's analysis of the most complete data identified for air ambulance transports of privately-insured patients, 69 percent of about 20,700 transports in the data set were out-of-network in 2017. This is higher than what research shows for ground ambulance transports (51 percent in 2014 according to one study) and other emergency services. Air ambulance providers that GAO spoke with reported entering into more network contracts recently, which could lower the extent of out-of-network transports in areas covered by the contracts.

While out-of-network transports may result in balance billing, the data GAO analyzed do not indicate the extent to which patients received balance bills and, if so, the size of the bills. In addition, as GAO reported in 2017, there is a lack of national data on balance billing, but some states have attempted to collect information from patients. For example, GAO reviewed over 60 consumer complaints received by two of GAO's selected states—the only states able to provide information on the amount of individual balance bills—and all but one complaint was for a balance bill over $10,000. Patients may not end up paying the full amount if they reach agreements with air ambulance providers, insurers, or both. The amounts of potential balance bills are informed in part by the prices charged. GAO's analysis of the data set with transports for privately-insured patients found the median price charged by air ambulance providers was about $36,400 for a helicopter transport and $40,600 for a fixed-wing transport in 2017.

The six states reviewed by GAO and others have attempted to limit balance billing. For example, the six states have taken actions to regulate insurers, generate public attention, or both. As required by recent federal law, the Secretary of Transportation has taken steps to form an advisory committee to, among other things, recommend options to prevent instances of balance billing.

March 20, 2019

The Honorable Roy Blunt
Chairman

The Honorable Patty Murray
Ranking Member
Subcommittee on Labor, Health and Human Services,
Education, and Related Agencies
Committee on Appropriations
United States Senate

The Honorable Rosa DeLauro
Chairwoman

The Honorable Tom Cole
Ranking Member
Subcommittee on Labor, Health and Human Services,
Education, and Related Agencies
Committee on Appropriations
House of Representatives

Air ambulances provide emergency services for critically ill patients, primarily in life-threatening situations. First responders call for air ambulances to transport patients from the scene of an injury or an accident to hospitals. Physicians also call for air ambulances to transport patients between hospitals when patients need higher levels of care, such as specialized trauma, cardiac, or stroke care.

The air ambulance industry, particularly as it relates to air ambulance helicopters, has seen numerous changes in recent years. In 2017, we reported that between 2010 and 2014 the median prices charged by air ambulance providers for helicopter transports approximately doubled, and the number of air ambulance helicopters grew by more than 10 percent.[1] We also found that various factors, such as the costs for and volume of transports, may play a role in air ambulance prices, but we concluded that an in-depth analysis of those factors is not possible due to a lack of data, including data on the total number of transports.

---

[1] Air ambulance helicopters are nearly three-quarters of all air ambulances. See GAO, *Air Ambulance: Data Collection and Transparency Needed to Enhance DOT Oversight*, GAO-17-637 (Washington, D.C.: July 27, 2017).

A health care billing practice known as balance billing may pose financial risk to patients covered by private health insurance who receive air ambulance services. Balance billing is when privately-insured patients receive a bill from a health care provider for any difference between the amount charged and the payment from the insurer for the service. For privately-insured patients who receive air ambulance services, balance billing can occur when they are transported by air ambulance providers outside of their insurers' provider networks, which means the providers and insurers do not have an agreed-upon payment rate.[2] For example, one consumer in North Dakota reported receiving a balance bill of approximately $34,700 for an air ambulance transport from Dickinson, North Dakota, to Bismarck, North Dakota, in November 2017. The air ambulance provider had charged $41,400, and the patient's insurer had paid $6,700, leaving a balance of approximately $34,700.[3]

There has been interest among federal and state policymakers and others in the issues of out-of-network air ambulance transports and potential balance billing. For example, the Secretary of Transportation has taken steps to form an advisory committee on air ambulance patient billing, as required by the Federal Aviation Administration (FAA) Reauthorization Act of 2018, which became law in October 2018.[4] Among other things, the committee is directed to recommend steps that states can take to protect consumers. The Joint Explanatory Statement accompanying the 2017 Consolidated Appropriations Act includes a provision for us to review air ambulance services.[5] In this chapter, we describe

- changes in geographic distribution of air ambulance services,

---

[2] Insurers have a group of designated providers with whom they have contracts to provide care to patients. Contracted providers accept negotiated payment rates with the insurer as full payment. Providers outside of that network—called out-of-network providers—do not have such contracts and have not agreed to a payment rate with the insurer. Instead, the insurer pays an amount according to what it allows for out-of-network services. Other types of health care providers may also send balance bills to patients.

[3] Source: North Dakota Insurance Department file number 105026. We do not have information on the extent to which the patient paid this balance. It is possible that the provider later discounted the bill.

[4] Pub. L. No. 115-254, § 418, 132 Stat. 3186, 3562.

[5] See Pub. L. No. 115-31, § 4, 131 Stat. 135, 137; 163 Cong. Rec. H3949, H3954 (Daily ed. May 3, 2017).

- the extent of out-of-network air ambulance transports and balance billing for these services, and
- what is known about the approaches selected states have taken to limit potential balance billing for out-of-network air ambulance transports.

For all three objectives, we interviewed officials in six states—Florida, Maryland, Montana, North Dakota, New Mexico, and Texas—that were selected to achieve variation among states in the growth in the number of air ambulance bases, the types of those bases (that is, helicopter or fixed-wing, which are the two types of air ambulances), the approaches taken in the state to limit balance billing, and geographic location.[6] We also interviewed officials from the three largest independent air ambulance providers, five national health insurers dominant in our selected states, and officials from the Centers for Medicare & Medicaid Services and the U.S. Department of Transportation (DOT).[7] To gain additional context, we also interviewed academic researchers and a consumer group who have examined the issue of balance billing, and we interviewed officials from local air ambulance providers and hospitals in three states (Maryland, Montana, and Texas) where we conducted site visits.[8]

To describe changes in the geographic distribution of air ambulance services, in addition to the interviews, we analyzed data in the *Atlas & Database of Air Medical Services* (ADAMS) on the locations of air ambulance providers' bases for 2012 and 2017, the most recent year for

---

[6] Some state approaches have faced legal challenges alleging preemption of federal law. We did not independently attempt to determine whether the states' approaches to balance billing were permissible under federal law, nor did we attempt to identify and report on challenges to these approaches in applicable state courts.

[7] As we have previously reported, there are three large independent air ambulance providers that dominated the industry and that reported operating 73 percent of the air ambulance helicopters in 2016. These are for-profit companies that handle both medical and aviation aspects of air ambulance transports and make business decisions, such as setting prices and determining contracts with private health insurers. Other air ambulance providers may be affiliated with hospitals. See GAO-17-637.

[8] Similar to our overall selection of states, we selected the three states we visited to achieve variation in the growth in the number of air ambulance bases, the types of those bases, the approaches taken in the state to limit balance billing, and geographic location.

which data were available.[9] We consulted with officials from the Association of Air Medical Services about limitations of the data, including that (1) these data are voluntarily reported by air ambulance providers with, according to officials, an estimated 95 percent of helicopter air ambulance providers and 90 percent of fixed-wing air ambulance providers in each year; and (2) the data include some air ambulance providers that do not offer air ambulance services on a full-time basis or that have a primary mission other than air medical services. We assessed the reliability of the ADAMS data by reviewing related documentation, interviewing relevant officials, checking for internal consistency, and comparing our results across data sets and to published sources. We determined the data were sufficiently reliable for the purposes of our reporting objectives.

To describe the extent of out-of-network air ambulance transports and balance billing for these services, in addition to the interviews, we analyzed private health insurance claims from FAIR Health for 2012 and 2017, the most recent year for which data were available, regarding the status of air ambulance transports as in- or out-of-network and the prices charged for those transports. FAIR Health is an independent, nonprofit organization that collects data for and manages a database of private health insurance claims data. The FAIR Health data set contains claims for around 24,100 transports in 2012 and 33,800 transports in 2017 from all 50 states and the District of Columbia, including claims from over 50 insurers in each year (including both fully-insured and self-insured plans). The data set accounted for 110.1 million covered lives in 2012 and 145.0 million covered lives in 2017.[10] This was the most complete data source we identified with data on prices charged for and the network status of air ambulance transports for privately-insured patients. However, the FAIR Health data may not be representative of all private insurers and therefore cannot be generalized. Our results on prices charged are based on all transports in the FAIR Health data. Our results on the extent of out-of-

---

[9] The ADAMS data show, among other things, the number and location of fixed-wing and helicopter bases in each state. The data are published as a partnership effort between the Association of Air Medical Services and CUBRC.

[10] This was 55 percent of the privately insured U.S. population in 2012 and 67 percent in 2017.

network transports are based on a subset of about 13,100 transports (accounting for about 58.6 million covered lives) in 2012 and about 20,700 transports (accounting for about 87.3 million covered lives) in 2017 with information on network status.[11] We assessed the reliability of the FAIR Health data by reviewing related documentation, interviewing relevant officials, checking for internal consistency, and comparing our results across data sets and to published sources. We determined the FAIR Health data were sufficiently reliable for the purposes of our reporting objectives.

We conducted this performance audit from October 2017 to March 2019 in accordance with generally accepted government auditing standards. Those standards require that we plan and perform the audit to obtain sufficient, appropriate evidence to provide a reasonable basis for our findings and conclusions based on our audit objectives. We believe that the evidence obtained provides a reasonable basis for our findings and conclusions based on our audit objectives.

BACKGROUND

Air ambulance providers use either helicopters or fixed-wing aircraft, as shown in Figure 1, depending on where and how far they are transporting patients.

- Helicopters are generally used for transports from the scene of the accident or injury to the hospital or for shorter-distance transports between hospitals. Helicopter bases may be at hospitals, airports, or other types of helipads, and a provider may need to fly from its base to the scene or a hospital to pick up the patient being transported. Air ambulance providers typically respond to calls for helicopter transports within a certain area around their bases in part to ensure appropriate response times.

---

[11] According to FAIR Health, two insurers did not report information on network status. This subset of transports represented 29 percent of the privately insured U.S. population in 2012 and 40 percent in 2017.

- Fixed-wing aircraft are generally used for longer-distance transports between hospitals. Fixed-wing bases are at airports, and the patient is transported by ground ambulance to and from the airports.

Air ambulance providers respond to emergencies without knowing patients' health insurance coverage, such as whether the patient has private insurance, Medicare, Medicaid, or no insurance.[12] According to our previous analysis of information from eight selected air ambulance providers, in 2016, Medicare patients received 35 percent of helicopter transports, privately-insured patients received 32 percent, Medicaid patients received 21 percent, uninsured patients received 9 percent, and patients with other types of coverage such as automobile and military-sponsored insurance received a small percentage.[13]

Relatively few patients receive air ambulance transports, but those patients who do generally have no control over the decision to be transported by air ambulance or the selection of the air ambulance provider, as shown in Figure 2. For privately-insured patients, this means they cannot necessarily choose to be transported by air ambulance providers in their insurers' network and can potentially receive a balance bill from the providers for the difference between the price charged by the provider and the amount paid by the insurer. This amount is in addition to copayments, deductibles, or other types of cost-sharing that patients typically pay under their insurance. Air ambulance providers are prohibited from sending balance bills to Medicare and Medicaid patients, while uninsured patients might be held responsible by the air ambulance provider for the entire price charged.

---

[12] Medicare is the federally-financed health insurance program for people age 65 or older, certain individuals with disabilities, and individuals with end-stage renal disease. Medicaid is a joint federal-state health care financing program for certain low-income and medically needy individuals.

[13] See GAO-17-637. Representatives of the providers we spoke to said that privately-insured patients accounted for the highest percentage of their revenue.

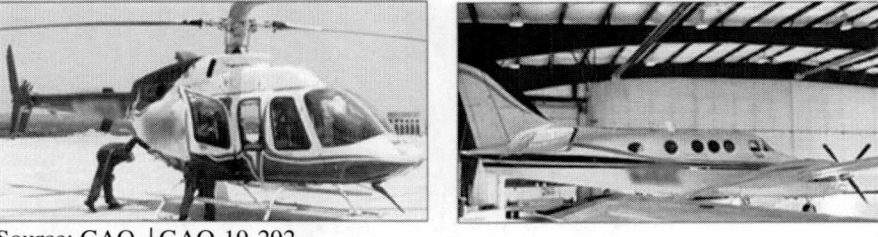

Source: GAO. | GAO-19-292.

Figure 1. Helicopter and Fixed-Wing Air Ambulances.

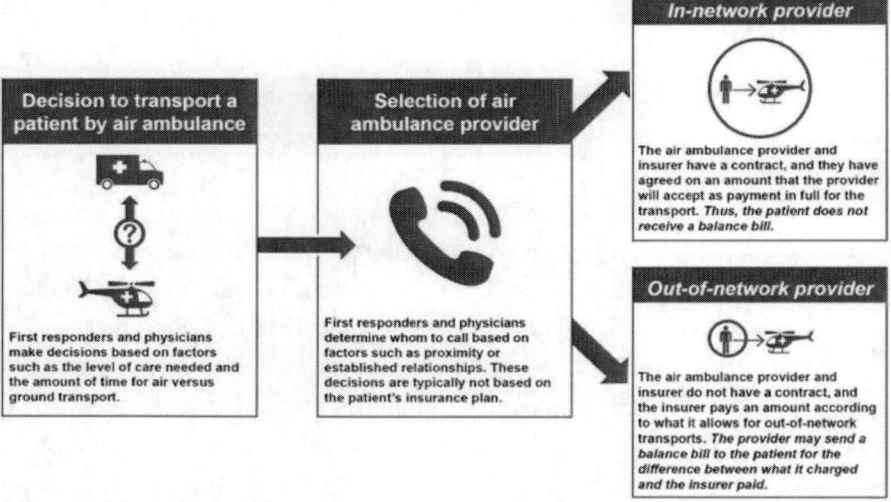

Source: GAO. | GAO-19-292.

Note: Patients may have cost-sharing responsibilities, such as copayments or deductibles, when transported by both in-network and out-of-network air ambulance providers. Also, patients may receive bills for the full charged amount if insurers determine transports were not medically necessary.

Figure 2. Air Ambulance Transports for Privately-Insured Patients and Potential for Balance Bills.

With many types of health care services, both health care providers and insurers have incentives to negotiate and enter into contracts that specify amounts that providers will accept as payment in full, thereby avoiding the potential for balance bills for those services. Insurers can offer—and health care providers may be willing to accept—payment rates that are much lower than the providers' charged amounts because the providers may receive more patients as an in-network provider. Furthermore, when patients are choosing insurance plans, they may consider how many or which providers are in-network, particularly for providers such as hospitals or certain physicians.

The emergency nature of most air ambulance transports, as well as their relative rarity and high prices charged, reduces the incentives of both air ambulance providers and insurers to enter into contracts with agreed-upon payment rates, which means air ambulance providers may be more often out-of-network when compared with other types of providers.[14] Decisions by first responders and physicians on which air ambulance provider to call are typically not based on the patient's insurance plan, meaning that being in-network may not increase air ambulance providers' transport volume. As a result, according to stakeholders we spoke to, if insurers offer payment rates that are much lower than the air ambulance providers' charged amounts, the air ambulance providers may be less willing than other health care providers to accept those payment rates. Furthermore, given the relative rarity of air ambulance transports, patients may not anticipate needing air ambulance transports and may not choose insurance plans based on which or how many air ambulance providers are in insurers' networks.

Approaches by states or the federal government to limit balance billing may target providers, insurers, or both. Examples of approaches described in research on balance billing include a cap on the amount that providers can charge or a requirement for insurers to pay the full amount charged by providers.[15] However, according to the research, targeting just providers or insurers can result in undesired outcomes. Capping the amount providers can charge could result in insurers that underpay for services, which could lead some providers to reduce service or exit the market altogether.

---

[14] As we have previously reported, costs to provide air ambulance transports are high and relatively fixed, such as costs for the staff required to maintain around-the-clock readiness. See GAO-17-637.

[15] For example, see Kevin Lucia, Jack Hoadley, and Ashley Williams, *Balance Billing by Health Care Providers: Assessing Consumer Protections across States* (Commonwealth Fund, June 2017); and Mark A. Hall et al., *Solving Surprise Medical Bills* (The Schaffer Initiative for Innovation in Health Policy, Oct. 2016).

Conversely, requiring insurers to pay the full amount charged by providers could result in providers that overcharge for services, which could lead to higher premiums charged to patients.

The authority of states to address issues related to air ambulance balance billing is affected by the following federal laws:

- *Airline Deregulation Act of 1978 (ADA):* A provision in this law preempts state-level economic regulation—i.e., regulating rates, routes, and services—of air carriers authorized by DOT to provide air transportation.[16] In general, courts have held that air ambulances are considered to be air carriers under the ADA's preemption provision, and courts, DOT, and state attorneys general have determined specific issues related to the air ambulance industry that can and cannot be regulated at the state level.[17]

- *McCarran-Ferguson Act of 1945:* This act affirmed that states have the authority to regulate the business of insurance.[18] For example, states may review insurers' health insurance plans and premium rates. In instances of balance billing, states can determine whether the insurer paid a provider in accordance with its policy for paying for out-of-network services.

- *Employee Retirement Income Security Act of 1974 (ERISA):* ERISA provides a federal framework for regulating employer-based pension and welfare benefit plans, including health plans.[19] Although states may regulate health insurers, ERISA preemption

---

[16] Pub. L. No. 95-504, § 4, 92 Stat. 1705, 1707 (codified as revised and amended at 49 U.S.C. §41713(b)).

[17] For example, as we have previously reported, the FAA regulates the aviation components of air ambulances, which includes maintaining and piloting the aircraft. States can regulate the medical component, which includes caring for the patient and, consistent with FAA safety requirements, the medical equipment carried on board. See GAO, *Air Ambulance: Effects of Industry Changes on Services Are Unclear,* GAO-10-907 (Washington, D.C.: Sept. 30, 2010).

[18] Act of Mar. 9, 1945, Ch. 20, § 2, 59 Stat. 33, 34 (codified as amended at 15 U.S.C. § 1012).

[19] *See,* Pub. L. No. 93-406, 88 Stat. 646 (codified as amended at 29 U.S.C. §§ 1001 et seq.).

generally prevents states from directly regulating self-insured employer-based health plans.[20]

In 2017, as previously mentioned, we reported on the increase in prices charged by helicopter air ambulance providers and on the lack of data on the factors that may be affecting prices charged.[21] We also found onlylimited information was available related to several key aspects of the industry, ranging from basic aspects—such as the composition of the industry by type of air ambulance provider, the prices charged by air ambulance providers, and the number of overall transports—to the more complex, such as the extent of contracting between air ambulance providers and insurers or the extent of balance billing to patients.[22]

Given DOT's authority to oversee certain aspects of the industry, we made four recommendations to DOT in 2017 to increase transparency and obtain information to better inform their oversight of the air ambulance industry: (1) communicating a method to receive air ambulance complaints, including those regarding balance billing; (2) taking steps to make complaint information publicly available; (3) assessing available federal and industry data to determine what information could assist in the evaluation of future complaints; and (4) considering consumer disclosure requirements for air ambulance providers, such as established prices charged and the extent of contracting with insurers. DOT has taken steps to respond to the first two recommendations, including adding information to its website describing how air ambulance complaints can be registered

---

[20] Such plans may be referred to as self-insured or self-funded employer sponsored plans. See GAO, *Employer-Based Health Plans: Issues, Trends, and Challenges Posed by ERISA*, GAO/HEHS-95-167 (Washington, D.C.: Jul. 25, 1995). Of the workers covered by employer-sponsored insurance in 2018, approximately 61 percent were enrolled in plans that were partially or entirely self-funded. See Kaiser Family Foundation, *Employer Health Benefits: 2018 Annual Survey* (San Francisco, Calif.: Kaiser Family Foundation, 2018).

[21] See GAO-17-637.

[22] As we reported in GAO-17-637, there is some limited data on the number of helicopter transports from requirements under the FAA Modernization and Reform Act of 2012, which directed FAA to collect certain specified operation data for the helicopter air ambulance industry and report this information to Congress by 2014 and annually thereafter. Pub. L. No. 112-95, § 306, 126 Stat. 11, 60 (2012). In May 2017, FAA provided its first submission, which contained a summary of data collected from helicopter air ambulance operators from April 1, 2015 through December 31, 2015.

and used by DOT. It has also listed the number of air ambulance complaints filed with DOT each month starting in January 2018—23 air ambulance complaints have been filed with DOT through November 2018. DOT has not yet acted on the remaining two recommendations.

AIR AMBULANCE PROVIDERS ADDED BASES FROM 2012 THROUGH 2017

Air ambulance providers added helicopter bases from 2012 through 2017, according to our analysis of the ADAMS data.[23] Specifically, there were 752 bases in the 2012 data and 868 bases in the 2017 data. When we compared the data for each year, there were 554 bases in both years of data (i.e., existing bases), 314 bases in the 2017 data only (i.e., new bases), and 198 bases in the 2012 data only (i.e., closed bases); the new and existing bases are shown in Figure 3.[24] This addition in bases also increased the total area served by helicopter bases by 23 percent.[25] Several air ambulance providers told us about their decisions to open new bases. For example, one air ambulance provider told us that one way it evaluates the need for a new base in an area is to ask hospitals in that area about the number of transports they typically require and the length of time it takes helicopters to arrive to pick up patients.

Along with adding helicopter bases, air ambulance providers also added fixed-wing bases from 2012 through 2017, according to our analysis of the ADAMS data. Specifically, there were 146 bases in the 2012 data and 182 bases in the 2017 data. When we compared the data for each year,

---

[23] We identified bases by the geographic coordinates in the ADAMS data, and some bases, such as certain airports, had more than one provider.

[24] The ADAMS data are voluntarily reported by air ambulance providers, and some of the changes in bases may be related to changes in which air ambulance providers reported data in each year. For example, after we completed our analyses, the Association of Air Medical Services identified 21 helicopter bases that were operational in 2012 but were not in the 2012 data due to provider underreporting. From 2012 through 2017, the average number of helicopters per base slightly decreased from 1.24 to 1.21.

[25] We calculated the potential area served by each helicopter base, in square miles, according to a 10-minute fly circle around the midpoint.

there were 114 bases in both years of data (i.e., existing bases), 68 bases in the 2017 data only (i.e., new bases), and 32 bases in the 2012 data only (i.e., closed bases); the new and existing bases are shown in Figure 4.[26]

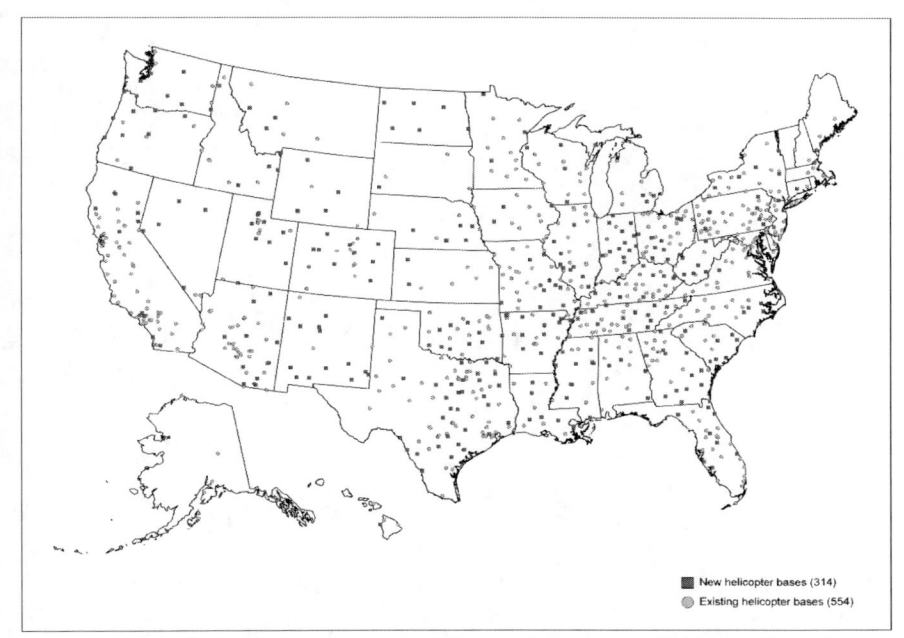

New helicopter bases (314)
Existing helicopter bases (554)

Soure: GAO analysis of data from the Atlas and Database of Air Medical Services (ADAMS). | GAO-19-292.

Note: Some bases, such as certain airports, had more than one provider. We identified 752 bases in the 2012 ADAMS data and 868 bases in the 2017 ADAMS data. Of those bases, 554 are in both years of data (i.e., existing bases), 314 are in the 2017 data only (i.e., new bases), and 198 are in the 2012 data only (i.e., closed bases, which are not shown in the map). The ADAMS data are voluntarily reported by air ambulance providers, and some of the changes in bases may be related to changes in which providers reported data in each year.

Figure 3. Helicopter Air Ambulance Bases, September 2017.

---

[26] The ADAMS data are voluntarily reported by air ambulance providers, and some of the changes in bases may be related to changes in which air ambulance providers reported data in each year. For example, after we completed our analyses, the Association of Air Medical Services identified 10 fixed-wing bases that were operational in 2012 but were not in the 2012 data due to provider underreporting. From 2012 through 2017, the average number of fixed-wing aircraft per base slightly decreased from 2.14 to 1.99.

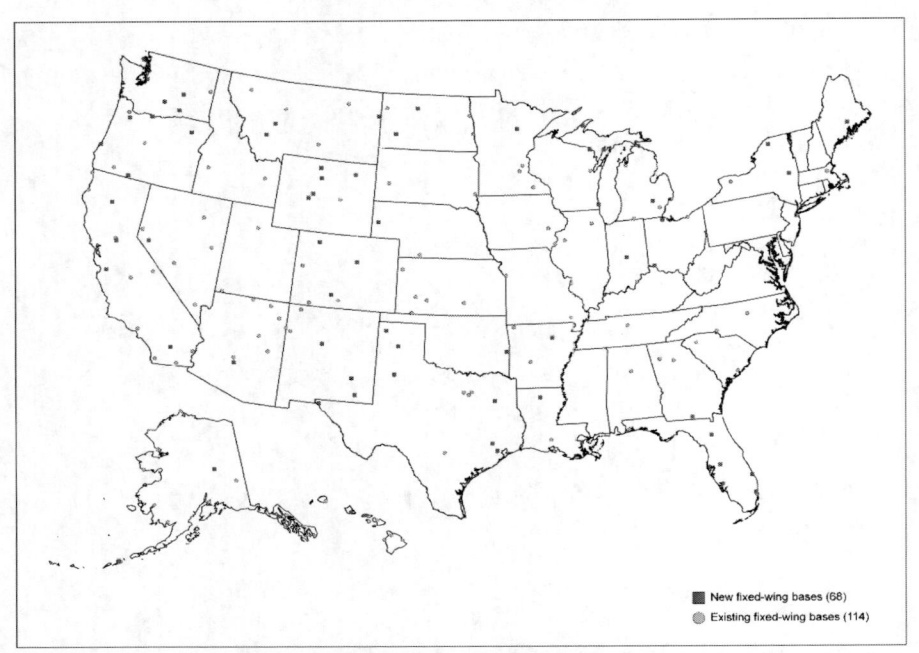

New fixed-wing bases (68)
Existing fixed-wing bases (114)

Soure: GAO analysis of data from the Atlas and Database of Air Medical Services (ADAMS). | GAO-19-292.

Note: Some bases, such as certain airports, had more than one provider. We identified 146 bases in the 2012 ADAMS data and 182 bases in the 2017 ADAMS data. Of those bases, 114 are in both years of data (i.e., existing bases), 68 are in the 2017 data only (i.e., new bases), and 32 are in the 2012 data only (i.e., closed bases, which are not shown in the map). The ADAMS data are voluntarily reported by air ambulance providers, and some of the changes in bases may be related to changes in which providers reported data in each year.

Figure 4. Fixed-Wing Air Ambulance Bases, September 2017.

Both the existing and new bases are more prevalent in the Western and Southern parts of the United States. Given that fixed-wing aircraft are used for longer-distance transports and that patients are brought to the base rather than picked up by fixed-wing aircraft, we did not measure the area or any changes in the area served by fixed-wing bases, which are usually airports. Based on our previous work, we further analyzed two trends related to where air ambulance providers have chosen to locate their new bases.

- *New bases in rural areas:* About 60 percent of the new helicopter bases and about half of the new fixed-wing bases in the ADAMS data were in rural areas. We previously reported that some helicopter air ambulance providers told us that the lower population density in rural areas leads to fewer transports per helicopter at rural bases.[27] They also said that, despite the lower population density, rural areas may have greater need for air ambulance transports. This may be due to, for example, the closure of some rural hospitals and the establishment of regional medical facilities, such as cardiac and stroke centers that provide highly specialized care.[28]

- *New bases in areas with existing coverage:* For just under half of the new helicopter bases in the ADAMS data, the area served overlapped with existing air ambulance coverage by more than 50 percent.[29] On one hand, according to some stakeholders we spoke to, the new helicopters may help enhance available services by, for example, being able to respond to a call if the existing ambulance resources are in use or otherwise unavailable.[30] On the other hand, as we have previously reported, some air ambulance providers told us that when helicopters are added to bases in areas with existing coverage, those helicopters are not serving additional demand.[31] As a result, the same number of transports is spread out over more

---

[27] See GAO-17-637. This report focused on air ambulance helicopters.

[28] As we have previously reported, out of 2,400 rural hospitals open in 2013, approximately 3 percent closed in the subsequent 4 years. See GAO, *Rural Hospital Closures: Number and Characteristics of Affected Hospitals and Contributing Factors,* GAO-18-634 (Washington, D.C.: Aug. 29, 2018).

[29] For helicopter bases, we calculated the potential area served by each base, in square miles, according to a 10-minute fly circle around the midpoint, and we determined the extent of overlap between the area served by each new base and the area served by all bases as of 2012. As previously mentioned, we did not measure the area served by fixed-wing bases, because fixed-wing aircraft are used for longer-distance transports and patients are brought to the base rather than picked up by fixed-wing aircraft.

[30] In addition, the ADAMS data includes some air ambulance providers that may not offer air ambulance services on a full-time basis or that have a primary mission other than air medical services. In some cases, a new base in an area with existing coverage may increase the number of hours that an air ambulance is available to respond to a call for a transport.

[31] See GAO-17-637.

helicopters, reducing the average number of transports per helicopter.

The FAA Reauthorization Act of 2018, which became law in October 2018, requires the FAA to assess the availability of information to the general public related to the location of heliports and helipads used by helicopters providing air ambulance services and to update current databases or, if appropriate, develop a new database containing such information.[32] This could provide additional information about base locations going forward.

AVAILABLE DATA INDICATE ABOUT TWO-THIRDS OF AIR AMBULANCE TRANSPORTS FOR PRIVATELY-INSURED PATIENTS WERE OUT-OFNETWORK BUT NOT EXTENT OF BALANCE BILLING FOR THESE SERVICES

In the FAIR Health data on air ambulance transports for privately-insured patients, about two-thirds of the approximately 13,100 and 20,700 transports with information on network status were out-of-network in 2012 and 2017, respectively. (See Table 1.) The proportions were similar for both helicopter and fixed-wing transports in each year.

Table 1. Out-of-Network Air Ambulance Transports for Privately-Insured Patients Analyzed

Year	All transports	Out-of-network transports	Proportion of out-of-network transports
2012	13,087	9,762	75%
2017	20,726	14,316	69%

Source: GAO analysis of data from FAIR Health. | GAO-19-292.

Note: Our results reflect the subset of transports in the FAIR Health data set with information on network status. The FAIR Health data set may not be representative of all private insurers.

---

[32] Pub. L. No. 115-254, § 314, 132 Stat. 3266.

The proportion of out-of-network air ambulance transports in the FAIR Health data set is higher than what research shows for ground ambulance transports and other types of emergency services. For example, one study found that 51 percent of ground ambulance transports in 2014 were out-of-network, and the same study and another one found that 14 and 22 percent of emergency department visits in 2014 and 2015 involved out-ofnetwork physicians, even at in-network hospitals.[33]

Air ambulance providers and insurers we spoke to confirmed that their proportion of out-of-network transports was high in 2017, but some also reported they have recently been entering into more network contracts.[34] For example, one of the large independent air ambulance providers and a national insurer entered into a contract that covered patients in five states as of August 2018. These contracts could decrease the extent of out-ofnetwork transports and balance billing in the future for these states.

Increases in the prices charged for air ambulance transports may exacerbate the financial risks related to balance billing for those with private insurance. In 2017, the median price charged by air ambulance providers for a transport was approximately $36,400 for a helicopter transport and $40,600 for a fixed-wing transport, according to our analysis of FAIR Health data.[35] The prices charged in 2017 were an increase of over 60 percent from 2012, when the median price charged was approximately

---

[33] C. Garmon and B. Chartock, "One in Five Inpatient Emergency Department Cases May Lead to Surprise Bills," *Health Affairs*, vol. 36, no. 1 (2017); and Z. Cooper and F. S. Morton, "Out-of-Network Emergency-Physician Bills—An Unwelcome Surprise," *New England Journal of Medicine*, vol. 375, no. 20 (2016). Some ground ambulance transports are from municipal providers, which may not enter into contractual agreements with private insurance companies.

[34] Some air ambulance providers and insurers provided data to GAO about the network status of transports by state across some or all of our six selected states. Nearly all state-level data from both providers and insurers showed that at least two-thirds of transports were out-of-network in 2017.

[35] Air ambulance providers, like other health care providers, charge standard prices regardless of insurance type. Prices charged for air ambulance transports have two parts: a service-level charge for the type of transport provided and a charge per mile that the patient is transported. Fixed-wing transports generally cover longer distances, and the mileage charge is therefore a larger portion of the prices charged. For example, in 2017, the fixed-wing mileage charge was over half of the total median charge based on a median charge per mile of $110 and a median distance of 204 miles. In contrast, the helicopter mileage charge was about one-third of the total median charge based on a median charge per mile of $242 and a median distance of 45 miles.

$22,100 for a helicopter transport and $24,900 for a fixed-wing transport. There is limited information on what insurers pay for outof-network services.[36]

While out-of-network transports may result in balance billing, the FAIR Health data we analyzed do not indicate the extent to which patients received balance bills and, if so, the size of the bills. In addition, as we previously reported, there is a lack of comprehensive national data about the extent and size of balance bills, and air ambulance providers are generally not required to report such data.

However, some states have attempted to collect information from patients about balance billing for air ambulance services. Therefore, to provide insights into potential balance bill amounts, we reviewed data on consumer complaints that two of our selected states had received about specific incidents of balance billing for 2014 through 2018.[37] Data for Maryland contained about two dozen complaints with information on the specific amount of balance bills, and those amounts ranged from $12,300 to $52,000. Data from North Dakota contained three dozen complaints with information on the specific amount of balance bills, and those amounts ranged from $600 to $66,600, though all but one amount was over $10,000.[38]

---

[36] Insurers' payment arrangements for out-of-network services vary and are detailed in individual plan documents, but a report from the Health Care Cost Institute, which included data from three, large national private health insurance insurers, cited the median payment these insurers paid for a helicopter transport was $15,600 in 2010 and $26,600 in 2014. We reported that while the data included approximately 40 million individuals with employer-sponsored insurance, patients in rural areas may be underrepresented. See GAO-17-637.

[37] Of our six selected states, Maryland and North Dakota provided us with complaint data that included information on the specific amount of individual balance bills. Other states provided more general information on the complaints they had received. Maryland's Office of the Attorney General, Health Education and Advocacy Unit, which mediates consumer complaints and works in conjunction with the Maryland Insurance Administration for state-regulated plans, provided data for complaints closed from January 2014 through April 2018. The most recent relevant balance billing complaint in the data was from September 2017. The North Dakota Insurance Department provided data for June 2014 through December 2018. The most recent relevant balance billing complaint in the data was from October 2018.

[38] The complaint data for both Maryland and North Dakota did not always include information on how much was ultimately paid. There were also additional complaints in the data for both states that lacked information on the size of the balance bills.

Given that providers may agree to reduce amounts that patients would otherwise owe or insurers may increase their payments to providers, along with limited national data, the extent to which patients actually pay the full amounts of balance bills received is also unclear.[39] Generally, officials from air ambulance providers we spoke to said that they first encourage patients to appeal to their insurers for increased payment. If these appeals do not fully address the balance bill, the providers may offer various payment options. For example, officials from one air ambulance provider said that it offers a discount of up to 50 percent off the balance bill if the patient pays the remaining 50 percent immediately. Alternatively, the provider requests detailed financial information—such as income, obligations and debts, and medical bills—to determine whether to potentially offer other discounts or a payment plan. This process can take multiple months, and officials from another air ambulance provider said patients who do not respond to letters and calls may be more likely to be referred to a collections process. Air ambulance providers we spoke with said that they use discretion on how much assistance to offer, and not all patients receive discounts after providing all relevant documentation. Even with discounts, according to data from some air ambulance providers we spoke with, the amount patients pay can still be in the thousands of dollars.

SELECTED STATES HAVE ATTEMPTED TO LIMIT POTENTIAL AIR AMBULANCE BALANCE BILLING THROUGH INSURANCE REGULATION AND PUBLIC ATTENTION

Four of our selected states attempted to limit balance billing through the regulation of insurers (Montana, New Mexico, North Dakota, and Texas). Additionally, four states have attempted to limit balance billing

---

[39] As previously mentioned, air ambulance providers are generally not required to report such data.

through education and public pressure on stakeholders (Florida, Maryland, New Mexico, and North Dakota).

Insurance Regulation

Four of the six states we selected—Montana, New Mexico, North Dakota, and Texas—have attempted to limit balance billing by air ambulance providers through the regulation of insurers, as shown in Table 2. Three states have faced challenges in federal district court related to whether their attempts to limit balance billing by air ambulance providers are preempted by the federal ADA. As of January 2019, the case in New Mexico was dismissed on procedural grounds, and the cases in North Dakota and Texas have been decided.

The hold-harmless requirement and dispute resolution process established by Montana's law is an example of how states are attempting to limit balance billing by regulating the business of insurance. Under the hold-harmless requirement, the financial risk for potential balance billing is transferred from patients to the insurer by limiting the patients' out-of-pocket costs to their cost-sharing responsibilities. However, according to state officials, the dispute resolution process established by this law had not yet been used as of December 2018. The requirement and process apply to transports for patients covered by Montana-regulated insurance plans.[40] It does not apply to transports for individuals in most self-insured plans subject to ERISA, nor does it apply to transports for individuals, such as tourists, covered by insurance plans regulated by other states. The stated purpose of the law establishing this process is to prevent state residents from incurring excessive out-of-pocket expenses in air ambulance situations in a manner that is not preempted by the ADA.[41]

---

[40] This includes group health insurance plans for Montana public employees and officers and for employees of the Montana university system.

[41] Mont. Code Ann. §§ 33-2-2301(2) (as added by S.B. 44 (2017)).

Table 2. Selected States' Use of Insurance Laws and Regulations that Aim to Limit Balance Billing for Air Ambulance Transports

State	Description
Montana	A 2017 state law imposes a hold-harmless requirement on insurers or health plans for charges pertaining to out-of-network air ambulance transports. That is, insurers or health plans assume responsibility for amounts charged to a covered person in excess of both allowed amounts and applicable cost-sharing amounts. It also requires the use of a nonbinding dispute resolution process, including a determination of the fair market price of the services provided, before an aggrieved party may pursue any remedy in court.[a]
New Mexico	Managed health care plans are required to make emergency care services available to covered individuals without requiring prior authorization and to ensure the provision of appropriate out-of-network services without additional cost.[b] New Mexico's Office of Superintendent of Insurance began applying these requirements to air ambulance services in 2017. A claim was filed in federal district court alleging that the application of this requirement to air ambulance providers was preempted by the Airline Deregulation Act (ADA). In December 2018, the court dismissed the claim for lack of subject matter jurisdiction.[c]
North Dakota	A state law effective in 2018 requires insurers to pay for out-of-network air ambulance transports at the average of the insurer's in-network rates for air ambulance providers in the state. This payment is deemed to be full and final payment by the covered person for the transport.[d] In January 2019, a federal district court concluded that this payment provision is preempted by the ADA.[e] The following month, the state Insurance Commissioner announced plans for North Dakota to appeal this ruling to the 8th Circuit of the U.S. Court of Appeals.
Texas	Payments for patients in the state's workers' compensation program made pursuant to applicable rate guidelines must be accepted as payment in full.[f] The Texas Department of Insurance Division of Workers' Compensation began applying this requirement to air ambulance services in 2016. A federal district court recently decided that the ADA preempts enforcement of workers' compensation rate restrictions on air ambulance services.[g]

Source: GAO analysis of information from selected states. | GAO-19-292.

[a] Mont. Code Ann. §§ 33-2-2302, -2305 (as added by S.B. 44 (2017)).

[b] N.M. Stat. Ann. § 59A-57-4 (1978); N.M. Code R. § 13.10.21.8.

[c] PHI Air Medical, LLC. v. N.M. Office of Superintendent of Ins., No. 2:18-cv-382, slip op. (2018 WL 6478626, D.N.M., Dec. 10, 2018).

[d] N.D. Cent. Code § 26.1-47-09 (as added by S.B. 2231 (2017)).

[e] Guardian Flight LLC v. Godfread, No. 1:18-cv-007 (D.N.D. order filed Jan. 14, 2019). In addition, the U.S. District Court for the District of North Dakota previously ruled that the ADA preempted enforcement of a North Dakota statute enacted in 2015 that created a "primary call list" of providers that were in network with health insurers covering a certain proportion of the state's population. The court found that the call list requirement was "precisely the type of state regulation Congress sought to prevent... in the ADA." See Valley Med Flight, Inc. vs. Dwelle, 171 F. Supp. 3d 930, 941 (D.N.D., 2016).

[f] Tex. Lab. Code § 413.011 (2017); 28 Tex. Admin. Code §§ 134.1(a), 134.203(d) (2017). Workers' compensation insurance generally pays benefits to an employee injured on the job regardless of fault or negligence, and the employee waives the right to sue for injuries.

[g] Air Evac EMS, Inc. v. Sullivan, 331 F. Supp. 3d 650 (W.D. Tex., 2018) (U.S. District Ct. granted injunctive relief, prohibiting state from enforcing rate restrictions).

Officials in Montana and North Dakota reported receiving fewer consumer complaints about balance billing after implementing their laws to limit balance billing. One reason for this decrease in consumer complaints, according to officials in Montana, was that uncertainty over the possible effects of the law has made most air ambulance providers more willing to enter into contract negotiations with insurers. The officials added that shortly after the law's enactment, a large insurer and a large air ambulance provider entered into a network contract. Additionally, another air ambulance provider in Montana confirmed that although it had provided out-of-network transports, it had not sent balance bills to patients since the law took effect. Officials in both states could not comprehensively report the extent to which instances of balance billing may have decreased in their state.

As required by FAA Reauthorization Act of 2018, the Secretary of Transportation has taken steps to form an advisory committee on air ambulance patient billing.[1] DOT issued a solicitation in December 2018 for applications and nominations for membership on this advisory committee. The committee is to consist of representatives from state insurance regulators, health insurance providers, patient advocacy groups, consumer advocacy groups, and physicians specializing in emergency, trauma, cardiac, or stroke care, among others. The Act directs the advisory committee to issue a report within 180 days of its first meeting and to make recommendations that address the following, among other things:

- The disclosure of charges and fees for air ambulance services;
- Options and best practices for preventing balance billing—such as improving network and contract negotiation, dispute resolutions between health insurers and air medical service providers, and explanations of insurance coverage;
- Steps that states can take to protect consumers consistent with current legal authorities regarding consumer protection; and

---

[1] Pub. L. No. 115-254, § 418, 132 Stat. 3562.

- The recommendations from our 2017 report, including any additional data that DOT should collect from air ambulance providers and other sources to improve its understanding of the air ambulance market and oversight of the industry.

Education and Public Pressure

Officials in three selected states—Florida, New Mexico, and North Dakota—have provided information to educate consumers and other stakeholders about balance billing for air ambulance transports. The Florida Office of the Insurance Consumer Advocate and the New Mexico Office of Superintendent of Insurance reviewed air ambulance transports in their states and issued public reports with recommendations to improve transparency and education, among other recommendations.[2] Florida's report, issued in June 2018, recommends that insurers and air ambulance providers improve transparency about the availability of in-network air ambulance providers in a given area and provide information about rate justifications and billing practices to help consumers anticipate potential out-of-network costs. New Mexico's report, issued in January 2017, recommends educating emergency room physicians and other health care providers about the impact of air ambulance bills on consumers and on how to select in-network air ambulance providers. Additionally, since 2017, the North Dakota Insurance Department has produced a publicly available guide showing which air ambulance providers are in-network with the three insurers in the state. This guide is part of the state's requirement that, for non-emergency transports, hospitals inform patients about the network status of air ambulance providers.[3] Although the three

---

[2] Florida Office of the Insurance Consumer Advocate, *Emergency Medical Transportation Costs in Florida* (Tallahassee, Fla.: June 2018); and New Mexico Office of Superintendent of Insurance, *Air Ambulance Memorial Study Report* (Jan. 2017). The Florida Office of the Insurance Consumer Advocate is part of the Department of Financial Services. As of November 2018, officials we spoke with said that neither state has implemented the recommendations listed in their report.

[3] N.D. Cent. Code § 23.16-17 (as added by S.B. 2231 (2017)).

large independent air ambulance providers we spoke with told us that non-emergency transports comprise only a small percentage of air ambulance transports, officials in North Dakota said some dispatchers and first responders reported using the guide to call in-network air ambulance providers when possible for emergency transports.

Finally, one additional selected state—Maryland—has increased public awareness of air ambulance balance billing, which has generated public pressure on air ambulance providers and insurers to encourage the two sides to negotiate contracts. The Maryland Insurance Administration convened a public meeting in September 2015 with the goal of raising public awareness about air ambulance balance billing in the state. The meeting involved statements from patient, air ambulance, hospital, and insurer stakeholders. One of the large independent air ambulance providers said that public pressure following the meeting, as well as subsequent engagement from the state insurance commissioner, were factors in securing a contract with a large insurer in the state.

AGENCY COMMENTS

We provided a draft of this chapter to the Department of Health and Human Services and DOT for review and comment. The Department of Health and Human Services told us they had no comments on the draft report, and DOT provided technical comments that we incorporated as appropriate.

James Cosgrove Director, Health Care

Heather Krause
Director, Physical Infrastructure Issues

In: Government Reports on Health Care …   ISBN: 978-1-53615-844-1
Editor: Eric Beyer   © 2019 Nova Science Publishers, Inc.

Chapter 2

DEFENSE HEALTH CARE: DOD'S PROPOSED PLAN FOR OVERSIGHT OF GRADUATE MEDICAL EDUCATION PROGRAMS[*]

United States Government Accountability Office

ABBREVIATIONS

DHA	Defense Health Agency
DOD	Department of Defense
GME	graduate medical education
IAB	Integration Advisory Board
MHS	Military Health System
MTF	military treatment facility
NDAA	2017 National Defense Authorization Act for Fiscal Year 2017
OAC	Oversight Advisory Council

---

[*] This is an edited, reformatted and augmented version of the United States Government Accountability Office Report to Congressional Committees, Publication No. GAO-19-338, dated March 2019.

WHY GAO DID THIS STUDY

DOD's health care system prepares medical personnel for wartime or humanitarian missions while providing health care to servicemembers and other eligible beneficiaries. It is responsible for ensuring that military servicemembers are physically and mentally fit to perform their missions and that it has an adequate number of medical personnel with the requisite skills and training to meet DOD's mission needs (operational medical force readiness). DOD uses GME programs to recruit and retain military physicians by providing specialized medical training through physician residencies and fellowships in exchange for active duty service obligations.

The NDAA 2017 included a provision for GAO to review DOD's GME oversight process, as detailed in DOD's July 2018 report to Congress. GAO assessed to what extent DOD's proposed oversight process, as outlined in its report to Congress, addressed each of the NDAA 2017 requirements. GAO compared DOD's process with the NDAA 2017 requirements; reviewed relevant documentation, such as minutes from planning meetings and charters for two new oversight entities; and interviewed DOD officials.

In commenting on a draft of this chapter, DOD did not fully agree with GAO's finding that the department had not developed plans to implement its new GME oversight process, citing as a basis certain preliminary steps it had taken. Based on the preliminary nature of these steps and other reasons explained in the report, GAO stands by its finding.

WHAT GAO FOUND

The National Defense Authorization Act for Fiscal Year 2017 (NDAA 2017) directed the Secretary of Defense to establish and implement a process to oversee military graduate medical education (GME). The goal was to ensure GME programs fully supported operational medical force readiness, and the NDAA 2017 included several requirements for the process. In July 2018, the Department of Defense (DOD) provided a report to Congress outlining its proposed GME oversight process, and GAO found that the proposed process addressed each of the NDAA 2017 requirements. (See table.) The process formalized practices that were already in place within the military services, while also establishing two new oversight entities—the Oversight Advisory Council and the Integration Advisory Board. These entities were chartered in late 2018 and report to the director of DOD's Defense Health Agency.

At the time of GAO's review, DOD had not developed plans for implementing the GME oversight process. DOD officials stated that they began their planning efforts in late January 2019 but were unsure how long this process would take.

March 28, 2019

The Honorable James M. Inhofe
Chairman

The Honorable Jack Reed
Ranking Member
Committee on Armed Services
United States Senate

The Honorable Adam Smith
Chairman

The Honorable Mac Thornberry
Ranking Member
Committee on Armed Services
House of Representatives

Comparison of NDAA 2017 Graduate Medical Education (GME) Oversight Requirements with Department of Defense's Proposed Oversight Process

NDAA 2017 oversight requirement	Department of Defense's proposed oversight process
(1a) Review GME programs to ensure, to the extent practicable, that such programs are conducted jointly among the military departments.	•The Oversight Advisory Council (OAC) will review the services' annual training plans to ensure GME programs are conducted jointly. •The Integration Advisory Board (IAB) will improve and formalize communication and collaboration, collect best practices, and make recommendations to maximize joint conduct of GME programs.
(1b) Review GME programs to ensure, to the extent practicable, that such programs are focused on, and related to, operational medical force readiness requirements.	•The OAC will assist the Defense Health Agency with optimizing military GME programs to improve readiness. •The IAB will review the services' annual training plans to ensure GME programs support readiness.
(2) Minimize duplicative programs.	•The IAB will assess GME programs for unwarranted duplication and identify areas for efficiencies.
(3a) Ensure that assignments of faculty, support staff, and students are coordinated among the military departments.	•The IAB will review annual reports on faculty and staff assignments and coordinate student placement through the existing Joint Services GME Selection Board process.
(3b) Ensure that military treatment facilities are used as training platforms when and where most appropriate.	•The IAB will ensure military treatment facilities remain the primary training platform for GME programs.
(4) Review and, if necessary, restructure or realign programs to sustain and improve operational medical force readiness.	•The IAB will review programs and performance data annually and will offer recommendations to restructure programs if necessary to improve readiness.

Source: GAO analysis of National Defense Authorization Act for Fiscal Year 2017 (NDAA 2017) and Department of Defense information. The numbering of the NDAA 2017 oversight requirements is for reporting purposes and does not reflect the full numbering in the NDAA 2017. | GAO-19-338.

The mission of the Department of Defense's (DOD) Military Health System (MHS) is to prepare medical personnel for wartime or humanitarian missions and to provide health care to 9.4 million servicemembers, their families, retirees, and other eligible beneficiaries around the world. The MHS is responsible for assuring that military servicemembers are physically and mentally fit to perform their missions. It is also charged with assuring it has an adequate number of medical personnel with the skills and training to meet DOD's mission needs— referred to as operational medical force readiness. DOD uses graduate medical education (GME) programs to recruit and retain military physicians by providing specialized medical training through physician residencies and fellowships in exchange for active duty service obligations. GME programs help DOD maintain the necessary pipeline of physicians for its military hospitals and clinics, referred to as military treatment facilities (MTFs), while also preparing its medical personnel to deploy.

The National Defense Authorization Act for Fiscal Year 2017 (NDAA 2017) directed the Secretary of Defense to establish and implement a process to oversee GME programs, with the goal of ensuring these programs fully support operational medical force readiness.[1] This provision included several requirements, such as ensuring that the multiple GME programs operated by each of the military services (Army, Navy, and Air Force) are conducted jointly.[2] The NDAA 2017 required DOD to submit a report to Congress describing its overall GME oversight process and included a provision for us to evaluate the process as outlined in DOD's report.[3] This review assesses the extent to which DOD's proposed GME oversight process, as detailed in its report to Congress, addresses each of the NDAA 2017 requirements.

To determine whether DOD's proposed GME oversight process addresses each of the NDAA 2017 requirements, we compared the process as detailed in DOD's July 2018 report to Congress with the requirements in

---

[1] Pub. L. No. 114-328, § 749, 130 Stat. 2000, 2242 (2016) (codified at 10 U.S.C. § 1094a).

[2] The Department of the Navy administers health care for the Marine Corps. The military services operate multiple GME programs covering 93 medical specialties.

[3] Department of Defense, *Report on Oversight of Graduate Medical Education Programs of Military Departments, Final Report* (Washington, D.C.: July 13, 2018).

the law.[4] In addition, we reviewed relevant documentation, including minutes from planning meetings, charters for two new entities established to oversee GME programs, and documentation of any meetings for these oversight entities. We also interviewed knowledgeable officials from DOD's Defense Health Agency (DHA) and the GME directors from each of the military services, among others.[5]

We conducted this performance audit from June 2018 to March 2019 in accordance with generally accepted government auditing standards. Those standards require that we plan and perform the audit to obtain sufficient, appropriate evidence to provide a reasonable basis for our findings and conclusions based on our audit objectives. We believe that the evidence obtained provides a reasonable basis for our findings and conclusions based on our audit objectives.

BACKGROUND

The military services' GME programs provide specialty training to medical school graduates who agree to an active duty service obligation. Through GME programs, military medical officers acclimate to the military while developing core competencies and critical wartime medical readiness skills, such as combat casualty care and treatment of injuries from explosive or biological incidents.

According to military service officials, specialty training through GME programs is an important recruitment and retention tool because it may encourage continued service beyond the fulfillment of the initial active duty service obligation. Programs are accredited by and follow the standards of the Accreditation Council for Graduate Medical Education, a

---

[4] DOD's oversight process will be implemented in the future; thus, we did not evaluate the effectiveness of DOD's proposed oversight process.

[5] DHA supports the delivery of health care services to beneficiaries of the MHS and has responsibility for shared services, functions, and activities of the MHS and other common clinical and business processes in support of the military services.

civilian organization.[6] In fiscal year 2018, there were 3,189 residents and fellows enrolled in DOD GME programs, training in 70 specialties, at MTFs.[7]

In addition to establishing a process to oversee GME programs, the MHS is in the midst of a series of other reforms that Congress also mandated in the NDAA 2017. These other reforms, which address aspects of medical readiness, may directly or indirectly affect GME programs.[8] For example, the NDAA 2017

- requires the establishment of a personnel management plan for certain wartime medical specialties, such as trauma surgery, anesthesiology, and emergency medicine;
- requires that DOD, in collaboration with the military departments, establish a process to define the military medical and dental personnel needed to attain operational medical force readiness; and
- requires DOD to implement measures to maintain the critical wartime medical readiness skills and core competencies of health care providers within the military services.

In addition, the NDAA 2017, as amended, transfers administrative and management responsibility for MTFs from the military services to DHA and requires DHA to assume responsibility for the policy, procedures, and direction of GME programs.

However, each military service's medical command remains responsible for recruiting, organizing, training, and equipping their medical personnel.

---

[6] The Accreditation Council for Graduate Medical Education is an independent, not-forprofit, physician-led organization that sets and monitors the professional educational standards for physicians.

[7] An additional 23 specialties did not have any residents in fiscal year 2018. The count of students only includes residents and fellows at MTF facilities, although residents and fellows may be trained in civilian GME programs as well.

[8] DOD's activities to implement these other requirements were outside the scope of our report.

DOD'S PROPOSED GME OVERSIGHT PROCESS ADDRESSES ALL NDAA 2017 REQUIREMENTS; IMPLEMENTATION HAS NOT YET BEGUN

We found that DOD's proposed GME oversight process, as detailed in its report to Congress, addresses each of the requirements for GME oversight outlined in the NDAA 2017. (See table 1.) According to DOD officials, the report formalizes processes used by each military service under the Joint Services GME Selection Board, a joint entity of the military services which places medical officers from the Army, Air Force, and Navy in internship, residency, fellowship, and non-clinical training positions.[9] As noted in the report, DOD established two new GME oversight entities—the Integration Advisory Board (IAB) and the Oversight Advisory Council (OAC)—which will carry out the oversight requirements and report to the director of DHA, who has the ultimate oversight responsibility. These new entities were officially chartered in late 2018 and include members from DHA and each military service, as well as other advisory members.[10]

According to DOD officials, the IAB began planning for implementation of the new oversight process in late January 2019.

DOD officials provided us with additional information about DOD's proposed GME oversight efforts for each requirement:

---

[9] According to DOD officials, at meetings of the Joint Services GME Selection Board, DOD officials also agree to any inter-service placements, which is the assignment of servicemembers to GME programs operated by services other than their own.

[10] For the IAB, these advisory members include representatives from the National Capital Consortium, San Antonio Uniformed Services Health Education Consortium, and the Uniformed Services University, among others.

Table 1. Comparison of NDAA 2017 Graduate Medical Education (GME) Oversight Requirements with DOD's Proposed Oversight Process

NDAA 2017 oversight requirements[a]	DOD's proposed oversight process[b]
(1) Review GME programs to ensure, to the extent practicable, that such programs are (a) conducted jointly among the military departments; (b) focused on, and related to, operational medical force readiness requirements.	•The Oversight Advisory Council (OAC) will review the services' annual training plans to ensure GME programs are conducted jointly. •The Integration Advisory Board (IAB) will improve and formalize communication and collaboration, collect best practices, and make recommendations to maximize joint conduct of GME programs. •The OAC will assist the Defense Health Agency with optimizing military GME programs to improve readiness. •The IAB will review the services' annual training plans to ensure GME programs support readiness.
(2) Minimize duplicative programs.	•The IAB will assess GME programs for unwarranted duplication and identify areas for efficiencies.
(3) Ensure that (a) assignments of faculty, support staff, and students are coordinated among the military departments; (b) military treatment facilities are used as training platforms when and where most appropriate.	•The IAB will review annual reports on faculty and staff assignments and coordinate student placement through the existing Joint Services GME Selection Board process (including inter-service placements).[c] •The IAB will ensure military treatment facilities remain the primary training platform for GME programs.[d]
(4) Review and, if necessary, restructure or realign programs to sustain and improve operational medical force readiness.	•The IAB will review programs and performance data annually and will offer recommendations to restructure programs if necessary to improve readiness.

Source: GAO analysis of the National Defense Authorization Act for Fiscal Year 2017 (NDAA 2017) and Department of Defense (DOD) information. | GAO-19-338

[a] The numbering of the NDAA 2017 oversight requirements is for reporting purposes and does not reflect the full numbering in the NDAA 2017.

[b] The director of the Defense Health Agency has the ultimate oversight responsibility.

[c] According to DOD officials, inter-service placement is the assignment of servicemembers to GME programs operated by a service other than their own.

[d] DOD officials stated that they prefer to conduct training at military treatment facilities, and, to the extent possible, they do so. However, if the military treatment facilities do not have the capacity, students may be assigned to civilian sites.

- *Ensuring GME programs are conducted jointly and program assignments are coordinated.* Establishing the two new oversight entities will help ensure that the programs are conducted jointly and that student assignments are coordinated.[11] The newly established IAB has the same members as the Joint Services GME Selection Board—including the military services' GME directors—and will continue the placement work, in addition to other oversight responsibilities. According to DOD's report, the IAB plans to meet at least three times a year and will be responsible for many oversight activities and for developing policy recommendations for OAC approval. The OAC plans to meet at least twice per year and ad hoc, as required, to review the IAB's work and evaluate recommendations.

- *Ensuring GME programs are focused on operational medical force readiness.* Under DOD's proposed oversight process, the new oversight entities—the OAC and IAB—will ensure GME programs are focused on operational medical force readiness. Members of the Joint Services GME Selection Board, who are now members of the IAB, explained that they consider their GME placement efforts to be aligned with readiness, in that they are filling the number of approved and funded GME slots allocated through the budgeting process. These officials told us that each of the military services is responsible for determining which training slots are needed to meet operational medical force readiness requirements. However, in February 2019, we reported that DOD's military services lack joint planning assumptions and a unified method to develop DOD's medical force requirements. As a result, DOD has not determined the optimal size and composition of the operational medical personnel it requires for achieving its missions. We recommended that DOD establish joint planning

---

[11] The NDAA 2017 requires DOD to coordinate assignments for support staff and faculty, in addition to students. According to DOD officials, DHA will ensure that GME programs have the needed faculty, in coordination with the military services. The report to Congress states that the IAB will annually review faculty and support staff placements.

assumptions and use these assumptions to determine operational medical force readiness requirements, and DOD concurred with this recommendation.[12] This information is important to ensure that GME programs—DOD's military physician pipeline—can support these readiness requirements.

- *Minimizing duplicative programs and restructuring or realigning programs as needed.* According to DOD officials, GME programs are regularly reviewed for unwarranted duplication and the need for realignment. DOD officials told us that they do not consider theircurrent GME programs to be duplicative and asserted that each GME program is justified and necessary to maintain current operational readiness of the military services. They noted that evaluating programs for unwarranted duplication requires a multifactorial approach that accounts for program accreditation requirements and interdependency of specialties, among other things. There are additional factors that affect decisions around restructuring and realignment, including the fact that GME programs are multi-year. Although there may be a shortage of qualified candidates in a specialty one year, there may be many qualified candidates the next, according to DOD officials. In late January 2019, the IAB planned to develop a formal process to evaluate unwarranted duplication, while accounting for the multiple factors it must consider, according to DOD officials.

- *Ensuring MTFs are used as the primary training platform.* MTFs, according to DOD officials, are always the preferred training platform for GME programs. Although MTFs were established for the purpose of providing medical care to eligible individuals, they also function as a readiness platform for teaching programs and skill sustainment, according to military service officials. We have previously reported that the Army and Navy prefer to train their physicians internally through military GME programs, while Air Force officials stated that using civilian GME programs allows

---

[12] GAO, *Defense Health Care: Actions Needed to Determine the Required Size and Readiness of Operational Medical and Dental Forces*, GAO-19-206 (Washington, D.C.: Feb. 21, 2019).

them to train the physicians needed to meet mission requirements, in light of the limited capacity of the Air Force's GME programs.[13] According to DOD officials, for MTFs to be the primary training platform, they must have the right patient load to provide sufficient training opportunities.

At the time of our review, DOD had not developed plans for implementing the requirements outlined in the report to Congress. Prior to signing their charters in late 2018, the IAB and the OAC had been meeting informally, and IAB members indicated that they initiated planning efforts to implement the oversight process in late January 2019. However, these officials were unsure how long these implementation planning efforts would take. These officials stated that their implementation planning efforts would include the identification of goals and potential risks for the mandated requirements, as well as an evaluation of the performance measures used by each of the military services. We have previously reported that leading practices for sound strategic management planning—establishing goals, developing strategies to achieve goals, identifying risks that can affect goals, and developing plans to assess progress toward goals—can help ensure organizations achieve their objectives.[14]

AGENCY COMMENTS

We provided a draft of this chapter to DOD for review and comment. In its written comments, DOD did not fully agree with our assessment that it had not developed plans to implement its new GME oversight process. (See app. I.) Instead, DOD said that it had developed a general

---

[13] GAO, *Military Personnel: Additional Actions Needed to Address Gaps in Military Physician Specialties*, GAO-18-77 (Washington, D.C.: Feb. 28, 2018).

[14] These leading practices for sound planning are derived from our prior work related to planning. See, for example, GAO, New Trauma Care System: DOD Should Fully Incorporate Leading Practices into Its Planning for Effective Implementation, GAO-18-300 (Washington, D.C.: Mar. 19, 2018) and GAO, Defense Health Care: TRICARE Select Implementation Plan Included Mandated Elements, but Access Standards Should Be Clarified, GAO-18-358 (Washington, D.C.: Apr. 13, 2018).

implementation plan and had started to implement the GME oversight process. To support this point, DOD made a distinction between general implementation and detailed implementation. DOD cited its informal meetings and the establishment of the IAB and OAC—which we acknowledged—as well as efforts conducted while drafting its report to Congress, as evidence of its general implementation efforts. The department also recognized that detailed implementation—which, according to DOD, would include a detailed plan and process for full implementation of the requirements in the NDAA 2017—would not begin until late January 2019. We did not distinguish between general and detailed implementation efforts nor did the DOD officials we met with during the course of our review. Instead, as cited in our report, we assessed DOD's planning efforts against our previously reported leading practices for sound strategic planning, which include goals, strategies to achieve goals, plans to assess progress, and the identification of challenges and risks. As DOD had not yet initiated formal strategic planning efforts for implementing its new GME oversight process, it could not demonstrate to us that it had taken these steps. Consequently, we could not report that DOD had developed plans to implement its oversight process.

DOD also provided technical comments, which we incorporated as appropriate.

Debra A. Draper
Director, Health Care

APPENDIX I: COMMENTS FROM
THE DEPARTMENT OF DEFENSE

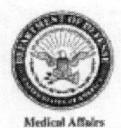

Medical Affairs

DEFENSE HEALTH AGENCY
7700 ARLINGTON BOULEVARD, SUITE 5101
FALLS CHURCH, VIRGINIA 22042-5101

February 28, 2019

Ms. Debra Draper
Director, Health Care
U.S. Government Accountability Office
441 G Street, NW
Washington, DC 20548

Dear Ms. Draper,

This is the Department of Defense (DoD) response to the GAO Draft Report GAO-19-338, "DEFENSE HEALTH CARE: DOD's Proposed Plan for Oversight of Graduate Medical Education Programs," dated January 30, 2019 (GAO Code 102875).

Sincerely,

Paul R. Cordts, MD

Paul R. Cordts, MD
Deputy Assistant Director
Medical Affairs Defense Health Agency

DoD Response to GAO Draft Report Defense Health Care: DoD's Proposed Plan for Oversight of Graduate Medical Education Programs (GAO-19-338)

The DOD **partially concurs** with this report.

The DOD responses to GAO findings are listed below with the requested changes (written in bold italic fonts for easy viewing).

1. GAO finding #1: GAO Highlights (p. 4 of PDF file): Bottom paragraph,
   "At the time of GAO's review, DOD had not developed plans for implementing the GME oversight process. DOD officials stated that they will begin their planning efforts in late January 2019 but were unsure how long this process would take."

   DOD response: Request change to
   "At the time of GAO's review, DOD ***had developed the general implementation plan and had started to implement the GME oversight process. DOD officials stated that they will begin their detailed planning efforts in late January 2019 to fully implement the oversight process.***"

   Justification #1:
   The final RTC was delivered to Congress on July 13, 2018. Balancing other statutory requirements, the J-7 Directorate and DAD-MA gathered the required background information from Service SMEs in order to inform the proposed process. As GME is new functional oversight for DHA, we have worked hard to recommend a process to the DHA Director that fully accepts the authorities outlined in NDAA FY19, as well.

The GME Working Group has met regularly since January 2017 to develop the oversight process, goals, and timeline for the RTC through a series of offsite meetings. This GME Working Group, which has functioned as the informal IAB, has been meeting on a near weekly basis since June 2018 to implement the oversight process described in the RTC. The IAB was officially chartered on November 26, 2018. The OAC also met on an ad hoc basis and was officially chartered on December 14, 2018. The implementation is continuing to ensure a smooth transition of the GME oversight responsibility through the chartered oversight advisory bodies, the IAB (O-6 or equivalent) and OAC (flag, SES), to DHA.

The Service Medical Departments and DHA have reviewed all GME residency and fellowship programs to determine readiness impact. The MILDEPs retain the responsibilities for determining requirements (number and specialty of physicians to be trained), as well as selection and assignment of GME military personnel (trainees and faculty).

DHA is establishing an interim central DHA GME Program Office to support the oversight function of DHA. The interim office will be become a permanent centralized GME office that works directly for DAD-MA. It also works directly with Service GME Directors, and MTF GME offices, in coordination with DHA J-7 Education and Training, the transitional Intermediate Management Organization (tIMO), and market leaders.

DHA continues to utilize MTFs as the primary GME platform with external/interagency partnerships, as needed, to ensure GME programs meet accreditation standards and meet validated military medical force operational requirements.

In addition, the IAB members have been working with Health Affairs for policy decisions by updating DoDI 6015.24, "Sizing of Graduate Medical Education and Program Closure Procedures". DHA is developing a DHA-Procedural Instruction to codify GME procedures and requirements outlined in the RTC on NDAA FY17 Sec 749.

The strategic plan to outline the goals has been completed and is described in Appendix B of the RTC. From 31 Jan 19 - 1 Feb 19, the GME IAB held an offsite to develop the procedures to minimize unwarranted duplication of programs and restructure/realign programs. With these new procedures, the GME IAB and OAC can evaluate progress toward the goals and risks to the goals annually.

2. GAO finding #2: Footnote 4 (p. 2 of report or p. 7 of PDF file)
    "DOD's oversight process will be implemented in the future;"

    DOD response: Request change to
    "DOD's oversight process *is being implemented;*"

    Justification #2: See Justification #1

3. GAO Finding #3: (p. 3 of report or p. 8 of PDF file)
    "...Accreditation Council for Graduate Medical Education, a civilian organization"

    DOD response: Request either
    a. Adding after the Accreditation Council for Graduate Medical Education *"(ACGME), ACGME is an independent, not-for-profit, physician-led organization that sets and monitors the professional educational standards essential in preparing physicians to deliver safe, high-quality medical care to all Americans,"* or
    b. Put the description of ACGME mentioned above as a footnote.

    Justification #3: For clarification of ACGME role

4. GAO finding #4: Subject heading (p. 3 of report or p. 8 of PDF file)
    "DOD's proposed GME...Requirements; Implementation Has Not Yet Begun"

    DOD response: Request change to
    "DOD's proposed GME...Requirements; Implementation Has *Started*"

    Justification #4: See Justification #1

5. GAO finding #5: (pp.3 and 4 of report or pp. 8 and 9 of PDF file – last sentence)
    "1) According to DOD officials, the report formalizes processes already in place under the Joint Services GME Selection Board..."

DOD response: Request change to
"1) According to DOD officials, the report formalizes *(in a joint fashion) processes already in place in each Service that culminate in* the Joint Services GME Selection Board..."

Justification #5: As stated, each Service GME Directorate has existing processes, the report synthesizes the Services' processes into one joint process.

6. GAO finding #6 (p. 4 of report or p. 9 of PDF file)
"The IAB will begin planning for implementation of the new oversight process in late January 2019."

DOD comment: Request change to
"The IAB has started implementation of the new oversight process and will meet in late January 2019 to develop a detailed plan and processes for full implementation of the requirements outlined in the RTC on NDAA FY 17 Sec 749."

Justification #6: See Justification #1

7. GAO finding #7 (p. 5 of report or p. 10 of PDF file)
"The newly established IAB has the same members as the Joint Services GME Selection Board and will continue the placement work."

DOD comment: Request change to
"The newly established IAB has *the Service GME Directors, who are members* of the Joint Services GME Selection Board, *and who will provide oversight in support of the OAC and DHA Director.*"

Justification #7: This is the more accurate description of IAB members.

8. GAO finding #8 (p. 5 of report or p. 10 of PDF file)
"...that DOD's military services lack joint planning assumption and a method to develop DOD's medical force requirements. As a result, DOD has not determined the size and composition of the operational medical personnel it requires for achieving its missions."

DOD comment: Request change to
"...that DOD's military services lack joint planning assumption and a *unified* method to develop DOD's medical force requirements. As a result, DOD has not determined the *optimal* size and composition of the operational medical personnel it requires for achieving its missions."

Justification #8: Each Service has a method of determining the medical force requirements as outlined in the report to Congress.

"The Department of Defense (DoD), through the Joint Staff, the Combatant Commands (CCMDs), and the MILDEPs, has a well-established process to identify force readiness requirements. The MILDEPs are tied intrinsically into that process, enabling them to define the military medical personnel requirements necessary to meet operational medical force readiness requirements, as required by section 721 of NDAA FY17. The process begins with the Defense Planning Guidance, and includes Defense Planning Scenarios and analyses of those scenarios by the MILDEPs to determine specific requirements to meet the proposed threats. The MILDEPs, in coordination with the CCMDs, are responsible for determining readiness requirements for Service members (Medically Ready Force) and the medical capabilities to support them. The MILDEPs provide the medical capabilities (Ready Medical Force). The goal of operational medical readiness is to meet and sustain DOD warfighting capability and provide the CCMDs the capabilities to meet mission needs."

9. GAO finding #9 (p. 5 of report or p. 10 of PDF file)
    "...**Minimizing duplicative programs**...DOD officials told us that they do not consider their current GME programs to be duplicative and asserted that each GME program is justified and necessary...to maintain operational readiness and to ensure adequate caseloads for medical residents."

    DOD comment: Request change to the first sentence of this section as
    "....maintain *current* operational readiness *requirements of the Services.*" Delete "and to ensure adequate caseloads for medical residents."

    Justification #9: The change reflects more accurately the IAB discussion.

10. GAO finding #10 (p. 5 of report or p. 10 of PDF file)
    Section "**Minimizing duplicative programs**... according to DOD officials."

    DOD comment: Request adding the following sentence at the end of this section:
    "In late January 2019, the IAB will develop a formal process to evaluate unwarranted duplication of programs to account for the multiple factors mentioned."

    Justification #10: The additional sentence gives Congress the next step which was accomplished in the IAB meeting in late January 2019. See Justification #1 for detail.

11. GAO finding #11 (p. 6 of report or p. 11 of PDF file) – First line of last paragraph
    "At the time of our review, DOD had not begun plans for implementing the requirements outlined in the report to Congress."

    DOD comment: Request change to
    "At the time of our review, DOD *had already started to implement* the requirements outlined in the report to Congress."

    Justification #11: See Justification #1

In: Government Reports on Health Care …   ISBN: 978-1-53615-844-1
Editor: Eric Beyer   © 2019 Nova Science Publishers, Inc.

Chapter 3

DRUG POLICY: PRELIMINARY OBSERVATIONS ON THE 2019 NATIONAL DRUG CONTROL STRATEGY*

Triana McNeil and Mary Denigan-Macauley

WHY GAO DID THIS STUDY

Over 70,000 people died from drug overdoses in 2017, according to the most recently available Centers for Disease Control and Prevention data. Overdoses have become the leading cause of death due to injuries in the United States, and most of these deaths involve opioids. GAO has a body of work on drug policy and ongoing work on ONDCP's efforts, including issuance of the National Drug Control Strategy. GAO also noted in its March 2019 High Risk report that federal efforts to prevent drug misuse is an emerging issue requiring close attention.

---

* This is an edited, reformatted and augmented accessible version of the United States Government Accountability Office Testimony Before the Committee on Oversight and Reform, House of Representatives, Publication No. GAO-19-370T, dated March 7, 2019.

This statement includes preliminary GAO observations on the 2019 National Drug Control Strategy and related findings from select GAO reports on federal opioid-related efforts. It is based on ongoing GAO work, two reports that GAO issued in March 2018 and October 2017, and selected updates on recommendations from these reports as of February 2019. For ongoing work and recommendation updates, GAO assessed the 2019 National Drug Control Strategy against statutory requirements, reviewed ONDCP and HHS documents, and interviewed ONDCP officials.

WHAT GAO RECOMMENDS

GAO has made prior recommendations to ONDCP, HHS, and other federal agencies to address drug misuse, including establishing performance measures with targets to better gauge progress toward achieving agency goals.

WHAT GAO FOUND

The Office of National Drug Control Policy (ONDCP)—responsible for coordinating and overseeing efforts by more than a dozen federal agencies to address illicit drug use—issued the 2019 National Drug Control Strategy on January 31, 2019. ONDCP describes the strategy as a high-level vision of federal drug control efforts, focused on prevention, treatment and recovery. The strategy designates one overarching objective to reduce the number of lives lost to drug addiction, and provides some description of federal agencies' activities, including steps to reduce the availability of illicit drugs. However, it does not include certain information required by law, such as annual objectives that are quantifiable and measurable, or a 5-year projection for program and budget priorities. This required information could help prioritize activities across federal agencies and measure progress over time, which previous GAO work has shown to be important for achieving results. GAO will continue to assess the strategy as part of ongoing work, and make recommendations as appropriate.

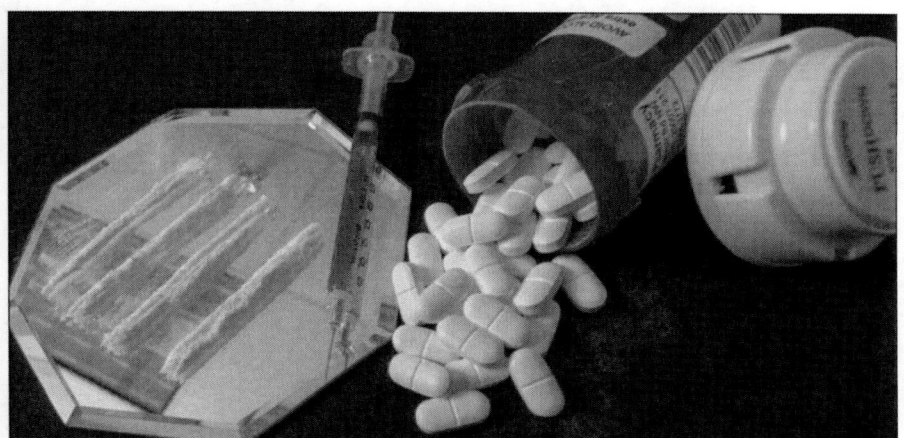

Source: GAO. | GAO-19-370T.

The lack of information in the 2019 National Drug Control Strategy on measuring progress toward its objective to reduce lives lost is particularly concerning in light of previous GAO reports. These reports found that individual agencies could do more to assess their particular efforts related to opioids. For example, GAO reported in March 2018 on five agency-specific strategies to combat illicit opioids, and also reported in October 2017 on the Department of Health and Human Services' (HHS) efforts to expand access to medication-assisted treatment for opioid use disorder. In these reports, GAO recommended, among other things, that federal agencies establish performance measures to better determine progress toward their goals. While federal agencies have taken some action to implement these recommendations, such as establishing performance measures for access to medication-assisted treatment, additional actions to measure the effectiveness of related drug control efforts would further help to gauge agencies' success, determine if new approaches are needed, and efficiently target resources.

Chairman Cummings, Ranking Member Jordan, and Members of the Committee:

We are pleased to be here today to discuss our ongoing work related to the Office of National Drug Control Policy (ONDCP), as well as two of our issued reports on federal opioid-related efforts that highlight the importance of assessing outcomes for the steps ONDCP and other agencies are taking to control illicit drug use and reduce deaths from drug overdoses.

While drug misuse in the nation is not a new phenomenon, the scale and impact of illicit drug use and prescription drug misuse has reached new levels, affecting individuals, their families, and the communities in which they live. Drug overdoses are at their highest ever-recorded level and, since 2011, have outnumbered deaths, respectively, by firearms, motor vehicle crashes, suicide, and homicide, according to the Drug Enforcement Administration. Over 70,000 people died from drug overdoses in 2017, according to the Centers for Disease Control and Prevention. Opioids—particularly highly potent synthetic opioids like fentanyl—are currently the main driver of these deaths.[1] The Council of Economic Advisers estimated that, in 2015, the economic cost of the opioid crisis alone was more than $500 billion when considering the value of lives lost due to opioid-related overdoses.[2] Primarily due to increasing rates of opioid-related deaths and opioid use disorder, the Acting Secretary of the Department of Health and Human Services (HHS) declared the opioid crisis a public health emergency on October 26, 2017.[3] We highlight these issues in our latest High-Risk

---

[1] There were more deaths in 2017 involving synthetic opioids than from any other type of opioid, according to the Centers for Disease Control and Prevention. Synthetic opioids are highly potent drugs manufactured to mimic naturally occurring opioids such as morphine. See GAO, *Illicit Opioids: While Greater Attention Given to Combating Synthetic Opioids, Agencies Need to Better Assess their Efforts,* GAO-18-205 (Washington, D.C.: Mar. 29, 2018).

[2] The Council of Economic Advisers, *The Underestimated Cost of the Opioid Crisis,* (Washington, D.C.: November 2017).

[3] A public health emergency triggers the availability of certain authorities under federal law that enable federal agencies to take certain actions in response. In September 2018, we reported that the federal government had used three available authorities since declaring the public health emergency to: (1) quickly survey more than 13,000 providers to assess prescribing trends for a medication used to treat opioid use disorder and any barriers to prescribing it, (2) waive the public notice period for approval of two state Medicaid demonstration

report, which we issued on March 6, 2019. In that document, we identify federal efforts to prevent drug misuse as an emerging issue requiring close attention.[4]

Federal drug control efforts span a range of activities including prevention, treatment, interdiction, international operations, and law enforcement. These efforts also represent a considerable federal investment. According to the President's fiscal year (FY) 2019 budget, federal drug control funding for FY 2017 was $28.8 billion. Multiple federal agencies have ongoing efforts to respond to the opioid crisis, including efforts to reduce the supply and demand for illicit drugs, to prevent misuse of prescription drugs, and to treat substance use disorders. As federal agencies engage in drug control efforts, ONDCP is responsible for, among other things, overseeing and coordinating the implementation of national drug control policy across the federal government.[5] These responsibilities include the Director of ONDCP promulgating a National Drug Control Strategy,[6] and assessing and certifying the adequacy of the National Drug Control Program agencies' budget submissions.[7]

In our testimony today, we will discuss our preliminary observations on the 2019 National Drug Control Strategy and how these observations relate to findings and recommendations from related, prior work. This testimony is based on our ongoing examination of ONDCP's strategies and programs. It is also based on two prior reports, which we issued in March 2018 and October 2017, that highlight the importance of assessing outcomes related to agency-specific efforts to address the opioid crisis.[8]

---

projects related to substance use disorder treatment, and (3) expedite research funding on medication development for opioid use disorder and overdoses. See GAO, *Opioid Crisis: Status of Public Health Emergency Authorities,* GAO-18-685R (Washington, D.C.: Sep. 26, 2018).

[4] Every two years at the start of a new Congress, GAO calls attention to agencies and program areas that are high risk due to their vulnerabilities to fraud, waste, abuse, and mismanagement, or are most in need of transformation. See GAO, High-Risk Series: Substantial Efforts Needed to Achieve Greater Progress on High-Risk Areas, GAO-19-157SP (Washington, D.C.: Mar. 6, 2019).

[5] 21 U.S.C. § 1702(a)(2). See also, 21 U.S.C. § 1702(a)(2) (2017).

[6] 21 U.S.C. § 1703(b)(2). See also, 21 U.S.C. § 1703(b)(2) (2017).

[7] 21 U.S.C. § 1703(c)(3)(E). See also, 21 U.S.C. § 1703(c)(3)(E) (2017).

[8] We are conducting our ongoing work in response to a provision in 21 U.S.C. § 1708a(b) that GAO routinely examine ONDCP's programs and operations, as well as in response to a

To develop our preliminary observations, we reviewed the 2019 National Drug Control Strategy, assessed it against relevant provisions of the Office of National Drug Control Policy Reauthorization Act of 2006 (ONDCP Reauthorization Act of 2006), and interviewed ONDCP officials. To perform our prior work, we reviewed and analyzed documents from ONDCP and other relevant agencies, reviewed relevant statutory provisions, and interviewed relevant agency officials. More detailed information on the scope and methodologies used to conduct our prior work can be found in each product cited in this statement. This statement also includes selected updates related to recommendations we have made in those reports. To conduct these updates, we reviewed documentation provided by agency officials in February 2019 about steps they have taken to address recommendations since the publication of each respective report.

We conducted the work on which this statement is based in accordance with generally accepted government auditing standards. Those standards require that we plan and perform the audit to obtain sufficient, appropriate evidence to provide a reasonable basis for our findings and conclusions based on our audit objectives. We believe that the evidence obtained provides a reasonable basis for our findings and conclusions based on our audit objectives.

BACKGROUND

More than a dozen federal agencies—known as National Drug Control Program agencies—have responsibilities for drug prevention, treatment, and law enforcement activities.[9] For example, the Department of Health

---

2018 congressional request. The two reports we reference are GAO-18-205 and GAO, Opioid Use Disorders: HHS Needs Measures to Assess the Effectiveness of Efforts to Expand Access to Medication-Assisted Treatment, GAO-18-44 (Washington, D.C.: Oct. 31, 2017). Other related work is listed in the Related GAO Products section.

[9] Currently under 21 U.S.C. § 1701(11), "the term 'National Drug Control Program Agency' means any agency (or bureau, office, independent agency, board, division, commission, subdivision, unit, or other component thereof) that is responsible for implementing any aspect of the National Drug Control Strategy, including any agency that receives Federal

and Human Services (HHS) has led efforts to expand access to drug treatment, and the Departments of Justice (DOJ) and Homeland Security (DHS) have taken lead roles in limiting the availability of illicit drugs through criminal investigations and prosecutions. The Anti-Drug Abuse Act of 1988 established ONDCP to enhance national drug control planning and coordination.[10] In this role, the office is responsible for (1) leading the national drug control effort, (2) coordinating and overseeing the implementation of national drug control policy, (3) assessing and certifying the adequacy of National Drug Control Programs and the budget for those programs, and (4) evaluating the effectiveness of national drug control policy efforts.[11]

Until its 2018 reauthorization, ONDCP had been operating under the provisions of the ONDCP Reauthorization Act of 2006 pursuant to annual appropriations acts.[12] In October 2018, the Substance Use-Disorder Prevention that Promotes Opioid Recovery and Treatment for Patients and Communities Act (the SUPPORT Act) was enacted and reauthorized ONDCP and a number of its programs.[13] The SUPPORT Act aims to address overprescribing and opioid misuse in the United States and

---

funds to implement any aspect of the National Drug Control Strategy, but does not include any agency that receives funds for drug control activity solely under the National Intelligence Program or the Joint Military Intelligence Program." In addition to ONDCP, these agencies include the departments of Agriculture, Defense, Education, Health and Human Services, Homeland Security, Housing and Urban Development, Interior, Justice, Labor, State, Transportation, Treasury, and Veterans Affairs, as well as the Court Services and Offender Supervision Agency for the District of Columbia, and the Federal Judiciary.

[10] Pub. L. No. 100-690, 102 Stat. 4181.

[11] 21 U.S.C. § 1702(a). See also, 21 U.S.C. § 1702(a) (2017).

[12] Prior to ONDCP's 2018 reauthorization, ONDCP had most recently been reauthorized by the ONDCP Reauthorization Act of 2006, Pub. L. No. 109-469, 120 Stat. 3502, through fiscal year 2010. The ONDCP Reauthorization Act of 2006 "repealed" the provisions related to ONDCP effective September 30, 2010. However, ONDCP continued to operate under the provisions of that Act pursuant to its annual appropriations acts. See Consolidated Appropriations Act, 2012, Pub. L. No. 112-74, 125 Stat. 786, 895-96 (2011), Consolidated and Further Continuing Appropriations Act, 2013, Pub. L. No. 113-6, 127 Stat. 198, 412 (2013), Consolidated Appropriations Act, 2014, Pub. L. No. 113-76, 128 Stat. 5, 195-96 (2014), Consolidated and Further Continuing Appropriations Act, 2015, Pub. L. No. 113-235, 128 Stat. 2130, 2344-45 (2014), Consolidated Appropriations Act, 2016, Pub. L. No. 114-113, 129 Stat. 2242, 2436-37 (2015), Consolidated Appropriations Act, 2017, Pub. L. No. 115-31, 131 Stat. 135, 340-41 (2017), Consolidated Appropriations Act, 2018, Pub. L. No. 115-141, 132 Stat. 348, 548-50 (2018).

[13] Pub. L. No. 115-271, 132 Stat. 3894 (2018).

includes provisions involving law enforcement, public health, and healthcare financing and coverage. Under both the ONDCP Reauthorization Act of 2006 and the SUPPORT Act, the Director of ONDCP is required to promulgate the National Drug Control Strategy and work with National Drug Control Program agencies to develop an annual National Drug Control Program Budget.[14] Prior to the SUPPORT Act, the Director was required to promulgate a National Drug Control Strategy on an annual basis, while under the SUPPORT Act, generally, the National Drug Control Strategy is required to be developed every two years.[15] ONDCP did not issue a National Drug Control Strategy for 2017 or 2018 despite the statutory requirement. Under both the ONDCP Reauthorization Act of 2006 and the SUPPORT Act, the National Drug Control Strategy is to set forth a comprehensive plan to reduce illicit drug use and the consequences of such illicit drug use in the United States by limiting the availability of and reducing the demand for illegal drugs.[16]

PRELIMINARY OBSERVATIONS ON THE 2019 NATIONAL DRUG CONTROL STRATEGY

As part of our ongoing work, we are reviewing the 2019 National Drug Control Strategy that ONDCP issued on January 31, 2019. Agency officials told us that they began preparing the National Drug Control Strategy in early 2018—prior to the enactment of the SUPPORT Act in October 2018. Officials stated that the National Drug Control Strategy was intended to respond to the requirements of the ONDCP Reauthorization

---

[14] 21 U.S.C. § 1703(b)(2) and (c)(2). See also, 21 U.S.C. § 1703(b)(2) and (c)(2) (2017).

[15] Prior to the SUPPORT Act, the Director of ONDCP was required to promulgate the National Drug Control Strategy which was to be submitted to Congress by the President not later than February 1 of each year. 21 U.S.C. § 1705(a)(1) (2017). Under the SUPPORT Act, the Director is required to release a statement of drug control policy priorities in the calendar year of a Presidential inauguration following the inauguration, but not later than April 1, and promulgate the National Drug Control Strategy which the President is to submit to Congress not later than the first Monday in February following the year in which the term of the President commences, and every 2 years thereafter. 21 U.S.C. § 1705(a)(1) and (2).

[16] 21 U.S.C. § 1705(b). See also, 21 U.S.C. § 1705(a)(1) (2017).

Act of 2006, which was the applicable law at that time. In light of ONDCP's stated approach, we based our preliminary analysis of the National Drug Control Strategy on the ONDCP Reauthorization Act of 2006. However, the SUPPORT Act retained certain similar requirements for the National Drug Control Strategy contained in the prior law.[17]

According to ONDCP, the 2019 National Drug Control Strategy provides a high-level vision of federal drug control efforts by focusing on prevention, treatment and recovery, and reducing the availability of illicit drugs. The 2019 National Drug Control Strategy designates one overarching strategic objective—to reduce the number of lives lost to drug addiction— and provides some general descriptions of federal agencies' activities. However, our preliminary observations related to the 2019 National Drug Control Strategy indicate that it does not include several pieces of required information, including the following:

- *Quantifiable and measurable objectives.* The National Drug Control Strategy was required to include "annual quantifiable and measurable objectives and specific targets to accomplish long-term quantifiable goals that the [ONDCP] Director determines may be achieved during each year beginning on the date on which the National Drug Control Strategy is submitted."[18] However, our work showed that the 2019 National Drug Control Strategy does not include this information. While it lists seven items that it designates as measures of performance or effectiveness, it does not indicate how they would be quantified or measured, or targets to be achieved each year. For example, one of the measures of

---

[17] Among other things, the SUPPORT Act requires the National Drug Control Strategy to contain: (i) comprehensive, research-based, long-range, quantifiable goals for reducing illicit drug use, and the consequences of illicit drug use in the United States; (ii) annual quantifiable and measurable objectives and specific targets to accomplish long-term quantifiable goals that the Director determines may be achieved during each year beginning on the date on which the National Drug Control Strategy is submitted; (iii) a 5- year projection for the National Drug Control Program and budget priorities; and (iv) a review of international, State, local, and private sector drug control activities to ensure that the United States pursues coordinated and effective drug control at all levels of government.

[18] 21 U.S.C. § 1705(a)(2)(A)(ii) (2017). The SUPPORT Act retained this requirement. See 21 U.S.C. § 1705(c)(1)(C).

performance relates to educating the public, especially adolescents, about drug use. However, it lacks information on how ONDCP would measure its efforts to educate adolescents, as well as targets ONDCP hopes to achieve, such as the number of adolescents educated or specific knowledge gains. Further, none of the seven measures has a baseline of current performance or annual targets, and four of the seven measures do not have associated timelines—which are important ways that results could be quantified. For example, one of the Strategy's measures of effectiveness is that evidence-based addiction treatment, particularly medication-assisted treatment for opioid addiction, is more accessible nationwide for those who need it. However, there is no information on the current level of treatment access, any targets for expanding access, or any associated timeline by which ONDCP hopes to achieve desired results.

- *Program and budget priorities.* The National Drug Control Strategy was required to include "a 5-year projection for program and budget priorities."[19] While the 2019 National Drug Control Strategy outlines several high-level priorities, including a top priority to address the current opioid crisis and its associated deaths, it does not include such a 5-year projection.

- *Specific assessments.* The National Drug Control Strategy was required to include specific assessments related to illicit drug use.[20] For example, the National Drug Control Strategy was required to include "an assessment of the reduction of illicit drug availability."[21] This assessment was to be measured by, among other things, the quantities of cocaine, heroin, marijuana, methamphetamine, ecstasy, and other drugs available for

---

[19] 21 U.S.C. § 1705(a)(2)(A)(iii) (2017). The SUPPORT Act retained this requirement. See 21 U.S.C. § 1705(c)(1)(D).

[20] While the SUPPORT Act does not contain the same specific requirements, it requires, among other things, that the National Drug Control Strategy include "[a] description of the current prevalence of illicit drug use in the United States, including both the availability of illicit drugs and the prevalence of substance use disorders." See 21 U.S.C. § 1705(c)(1)(K).

[21] 21 U.S.C. § 1705(a)(2)(A)(vi) (2017).

consumption in the United States; the amount of marijuana, cocaine, heroin, methamphetamine, ecstasy, and precursor chemicals and other drugs entering the United States; and the number of illicit manufacturing laboratories seized and destroyed as well as the number of hectares of marijuana, poppy, and coca cultivated and destroyed domestically and in other countries. The 2019 National Drug Control Strategy does not include this information. In addition, the National Drug Control Strategy was required to include "an assessment of the reduction of the consequences of illicit drug use and availability."[22] This assessment was to include the burden illicit drug users placed on hospital emergency departments; the annual national health care cost of illicit drug use; and the extent of illicit drug-related crime and criminal activity. Similarly, the 2019 National Drug Control Strategy does not include this information.

- *Performance measurement system.* The ONDCP Director was required to submit "as part of the National Drug Control Strategy a description of a national drug control performance measurement system."[23] Among other things, this system was to describe the sources of information and data that would be used for each performance measure incorporated into the performance measurement system. This system was also to coordinate the development and implementation of national drug control data

---

[22] U.S.C. § 1705(a)(2)(A)(vii) (2017).

[23] 21 U.S.C. § 1705(c) (2017). While the SUPPORT Act does not contain the same specific requirements, it does require the development of an annual national drug control assessment. Specifically, the Director is required to submit to the President, Congress, and the appropriate congressional committees, "a report assessing the progress of each National Drug Control Program Agency toward achieving each goal, objective, and target contained in the National Drug Control Strategy applicable to the prior fiscal year" not later than the first Monday in February of each year. In addition, the Director is to include in the annual assessment (i) a summary of each evaluation received from the head of each National Drug Control Program Agency; (ii) a summary of the progress each National Drug Control Program Agency toward the National Drug Control Strategy goals of the agency using the performance measures developed for the agency; (iii) an assessment of the effectiveness of each National Drug Control Program Agency and program in achieving the National Drug Control Strategy for the previous year; and (iv) the assessments required are to be based on the Performance Measurement System. 21 U.S.C. § 1705(g)(1) and (3).

collection and reporting systems to support policy formulation and performance measurement. Further, the system was to monitor consistency across the drug-related goals and objectives of the National Drug Control Program agencies and ensure that each agency's goals and budgets support are fully consistent with the National Drug Control Strategy. The 2019 National Drug Control Strategy does not contain a description of such a national drug control performance measurement system.

- As part of our ongoing work, we also asked ONDCP for information regarding how ONDCP officials determined the adequacy of National Drug Control Program agencies' budget submissions without a National Drug Control Strategy in effect for 2017 and 2018. The National Drug Control Program Budget is to provide information on federal drug control funding requested by the executive branch to implement the National Drug Control Strategy. National Drug Control Program agencies are required to submit to ONDCP the portion of their annual budget requests dedicated to drug control activity undertaken by the department, agency, or program. Agencies are to prepare these as part of their overall budget submission to the Office of Management and Budget for inclusion in the President's annual budget request. ONDCP is required to review and certify whether these budgets are sufficient to support the relevant goals and objectives outlined in the National Drug Control Strategy and then include these budgets in the consolidated National Drug Control Program Budget, which the President issues alongside his budget each year. As of March 4, 2019, ONDCP had not provided information on how it accomplished the required determination. In addition, as of March 4, 2019, the President's FY 2020 budget, and the accompanying National Drug Control Program Budget, had not been released. We will continue to consider ONDCP's activities in this area as part of our ongoing work.
- As part of our ongoing work, we will also discuss the 2019 National Drug Control Strategy with ONDCP and plan to examine

how ONDCP intends to address additional requirements in the SUPPORT Act. The lack of information in the 2019 National Drug Control Strategy on assessing progress toward its objective to reduce lives lost reflects findings in our previous reports. Our prior work in general, and our work on federal drug control efforts in particular, has consistently emphasized the importance of setting clear priorities through measurable and quantifiable goals, and assessing progress toward those goals over time, in order to achieve results.[24] For example:

- In March 2018, we reported on federal agencies' efforts—including those of ONDCP—to limit the availability of and enhance their response to illicit opioids, such as heroin and fentanyl.[25] We reviewed five strategies related to combating illicit opioids and determined that only one included outcome-oriented performance measures that aim to assess the effectiveness of its efforts— ONDCP's Heroin Availability Reduction Plan (HARP).[26] In contrast, we found that ONDCP's High Intensity Drug Trafficking Areas (HIDTA) programs' Heroin Response Strategy did not include any outcome-oriented performance measures.[27] Outcome

---

[24] For example, see GAO, Managing for Results: Government-wide Actions Needed to Improve Agencies' Use of Performance Information in Decision Making, GAO-18-609SP, (Washington, D.C.: Sep. 5, 2018); GAO, Managing for Results: Further Progress Made in Implementing the GPRA Modernization Act, but Additional Actions Needed to Address Pressing Governance Challenges, GAO-17-775, (Washington, D.C.: Sep. 29, 2017); GAO, Managing for Results: Enhancing Agency Use of Performance Information for Management Decision Making, GAO-05-927, (Washington, D.C.: Sep. 9, 2005); and GAO, Results-Oriented Government: GPRA Has Established a Solid Foundation for Achieving Greater Results, GAO-04-38, (Washington, D.C.: Mar. 10, 2004).

[25] GAO-18-205.

[26] The HARP, implemented in 2016, aims to provide a roadmap to guide and synchronize interagency activities, performed through ONDCP's National Heroin Coordination Group, to reduce the supply of drugs such as heroin and fentanyl in the U.S. market. See GAO-18-205 for more information.

[27] The HIDTA program, which is administered by ONDCP, provides assistance to federal, state, local, and tribal law enforcement agencies operating in areas determined to be critical drug-trafficking regions of the United States. The Heroin Response Strategy, started in 2015, seeks to bring public health and public safety partners together at the federal, state, and local level to reduce drug overdose fatalities and disrupt trafficking in illicit opioids. Like the Heroin Response Strategy, the other three strategies we reviewed did not include any outcome-oriented performance measures. These strategies were the (1) Organized Crime Drug Enforcement Task Forces' National Heroin Initiative, (2) Department of Justice and

measures address the results of programs and services, such as reductions in overdose deaths, and they can help in assessing the status of program operations, identifying areas that need improvement, and ensuring accountability for results. Among other things, we recommended in March 2018 that ONDCP coordinate with the HIDTAs to establish outcome-oriented performance measures to assess progress towards the goals set out in the Heroin Response Strategy. While ONDCP neither agreed nor disagreed with our recommendation, ONDCP told us in June 2018 that they had engaged with leaders from the HIDTAs participating in the Heroin Response Strategy to develop performance measures, including some outcome performance measures. As of March 4, 2019, this recommendation has not yet been addressed and ONDCP has not provided additional information on these efforts. We continue to believe that establishing these measures would enhance the HIDTAs' ability to assess whether these efforts are producing intended results.

- In October 2017, we reported on HHS's efforts to reduce the prevalence of opioid misuse and the fatalities associated with it by expanding access to medication-assisted treatment (MAT) for opioid use disorder.[28] These efforts included four grant programs that focus on expanding access to MAT in various settings (including rural primary care practices and health centers) and implementing regulatory and statutory changes that expanded treatment capacity by increasing patient limits for a MAT medication—buprenorphine—and by expanding the types of practitioners who can prescribe it in an office-based setting. We found that HHS had not established performance measures with targets that would

---

U.S. Attorneys Offices' Strategies to Address the Opioid Epidemic, and (3) Drug Enforcement Administration's 360 Strategy. See GAO-18-205 for more information.

[28] GAO-18-44. For those who misuse or are addicted to opioids—a condition known as opioid use disorder—research shows that MAT is an effective treatment. MAT for opioid use disorder combines behavioral therapy and the use of certain medications (methadone, buprenorphine, and naltrexone) and has been shown to reduce opioid use and increase treatment retention compared to abstinence-based treatment, where patients are treated without medication.

specify the results that HHS hoped to achieve through its efforts, and by when. We concluded that without this information, HHS would not have an effective means to determine whether its efforts are helping to expand access to MAT or whether new approaches are needed.[29] Among other things, we recommended that HHS establish performance measures with targets related to expanding access to MAT for opioid use disorders. HHS concurred with the recommendation and in February 2019, provided information that the agency had established performance measures with targets to increase the number of prescriptions for certain MAT medications, one of the potential ways to measure access to MAT. However, the recommendation has not yet been fully addressed, in part because HHS did not provide information on measures related to the treatment capacity of providers who prescribe or administer MAT medications, which HHS had identified as another way to measure access. We continue to believe that fully implementing this recommendation will help ensure that invested resources in the program are yielding intended results.

As our prior work shows, using data—such as information collected by performance measures and findings from program evaluations and research studies—to drive decision-making can help federal agencies improve program implementation, identify and correct problems, and make other management decisions.[30] Although agencies may struggle to effectively use this approach, regular performance reviews and evidence-based policy tools can help them incorporate performance information into federal decision-making. Without effective long-term plans, such as a national

---

[29] As we reported in GAO-18-44, gauging this progress is particularly important given the large nationwide gap between the total number of individuals who could benefit from MAT and the limited number who can currently access it based on provider availability.

[30] GAO-18-609SP. In addition, the Government Performance and Results Act of 1993, Pub. L. No. 103-62, 107 Stat. 285, sets out the performance planning and reporting framework. The GPRA Modernization Act of 2010, Pub. L. No. 111-352, 124 Stat. 3866 (2011), enhanced the Government Performance and Results Act by providing important tools that can help decision makers address challenges facing the federal government, help resolve longstanding performance and management problems, and provide greater accountability for results.

strategy, that clearly articulate goals and objectives and without specific measures to track performance, federal agencies cannot fully assess whether taxpayer dollars are invested in ways that will achieve desired outcomes. ONDCP's responsibility to develop the National Drug Control Strategy and coordinate among federal agencies offers the agency an important opportunity to guide federal activities to address the unprecedented number of drug overdose deaths. We are continuing with ongoing and planned work to monitor and assess federal drug control efforts.

Chairman Cummings, Ranking Member Jordan, and Members of the Committee, this concludes our prepared statement. We would be happy to respond to any questions you may have at this time.

In: Government Reports on Health Care ...   ISBN: 978-1-53615-844-1
Editor: Eric Beyer   © 2019 Nova Science Publishers, Inc.

Chapter 4

MEDICARE AND MEDICAID: CMS SHOULD ASSESS DOCUMENTATION NECESSARY TO IDENTIFY IMPROPER PAYMENTS[*]

United States Government Accountability Office

ABBREVIATIONS

CERT	Comprehensive Error Rate Testing
CMS	Centers for Medicare & Medicaid Services
DME	durable medical equipment
FFS	fee-for-service
HHS	Department of Health and Human Services
HHS-OIG	Department of Health and Human Services' Office of the Inspector General
IPIA	Improper Payments Information Act of 2002
IRR	interrater reliability

[*] This is an edited, reformatted and augmented version of United States Government Accountability Office; Congressional Addressees, Publication No. GAO-19-277, dated March 2019.

OMB   Office of Management and Budget
PERM   Payment Error Rate Measurement

WHY GAO DID THIS STUDY

In fiscal year 2017, Medicare FFS had an estimated $23.2 billion in improper payments due to insufficient documentation, while Medicaid FFS had $4.3 billion—accounting for most of the programs' estimated FFS medical review improper payments. Medicare FFS coverage policies are generally national, and the program directly pays providers, while Medicaid provides states flexibility to design coverage policies, and the federal government and states share in program financing.

Among other things, GAO examined: (1) Medicare and Medicaid documentation requirements and factors that contribute to improper payments due to insufficient documentation; and (2) the extent to which Medicaid reviews provide states with actionable information. GAO reviewed Medicare and Medicaid documentation requirements and improper payment data for fiscal years 2005 through 2017, and interviewed officials from CMS, CMS contractors, and six state Medicaid programs. GAO selected the states based on, among other criteria, variation in estimated state improper payment rates, and FFS spending and enrollment.

WHAT GAO RECOMMENDS

GAO is making four recommendations to CMS, including that CMS assess and ensure the effectiveness of Medicare and Medicaid documentation requirements, and that CMS take steps to ensure Medicaid's medical reviews effectively address causes of improper payments and result in appropriate corrective actions. CMS concurred with three recommendations, but did not concur with the recommendation on

Medicaid medical reviews. GAO maintains that this recommendation is valid as discussed in this chapter.

WHAT GAO FOUND

The Centers for Medicare & Medicaid Services (CMS) uses estimates of improper payments to help identify the causes and extent of Medicare and Medicaid program risks and develop strategies to protect the integrity of the programs. CMS estimates Medicare and Medicaid fee-for-service (FFS) improper payments, in part, by conducting medical reviews— reviews of provider-submitted medical record documentation to determine whether the services were medically necessary and complied with coverage policies. Payments for services not sufficiently documented are considered improper payments. In recent years, CMS estimated substantially more improper payments in Medicare, relative to Medicaid, primarily due to insufficient documentation (see figure).

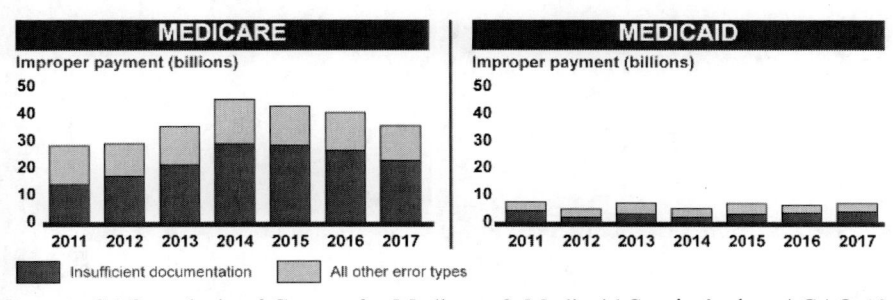

Source: GAO analysis of Centers for Medicare & Medicaid Service's data. | GAO-19-277.

Estimated Improper Payments Identified through Medical Review in Medicare and Medicaid Fee-for-service, Fiscal Years 2011-2017.

For certain services, Medicare generally has more extensive documentation requirements than Medicaid. For example, Medicare requires additional documentation for services that involve physician referrals, while Medicaid requirements vary by state and may rely on other mechanisms—such as requiring approval before services are provided—to ensure compliance with coverage policies. Although Medicare and Medicaid pay for similar services, the same documentation for the same service can be sufficient in one program but not the other. The substantial variation in the programs' improper payments raises questions about how well the programs' documentation requirements help identify causes of program risks. As a result, CMS may not have the information it needs to effectively address program risks and direct program integrity efforts.

CMS's Medicaid medical reviews may not provide the robust state-specific information needed to identify causes of improper payments and address program risks. In fiscal year 2017, CMS medical reviews identified fewer than 10 improper payments in more than half of all states. CMS directs states to develop corrective actions specific to each identified improper payment. However, because individual improper payments may not be representative of the causes of improper payments in a state, the resulting corrective actions may not effectively address program risks and may misdirect state program integrity efforts. Augmenting medical reviews with other sources of information, such as state auditor findings, is one option to better ensure that corrective actions address program risks.

March 27, 2019

Congressional Addressees

Medicare and Medicaid provide health insurance coverage to nearly 120 million Americans, with combined annual expenditures that exceeded $1 trillion in fiscal year 2017.[1] We have designated Medicare and Medicaid high-risk programs in part because their size and complexity make them vulnerable to improper payments—payments that should not

---

[1] Medicare is the federally financed health insurance program for persons aged 65 and over, certain individuals with disabilities, and individuals with end-stage renal disease. Medicaid is a joint federal-state program that finances health care for low-income and medically needy individuals.

have been made or were made in incorrect amounts based on program requirements.[2]

Medicare and Medicaid provide health coverage through different mechanisms, including fee-for-service (FFS), in which individual health care providers are paid for each service delivered.[3] In fiscal year 2017, Medicare FFS spending was an estimated $381 billion, and combined federal and state spending for Medicaid FFS was an estimated $320 billion. In the same year, estimated Medicare FFS improper payments were $36.2 billion and estimated Medicaid FFS improper payments were $41.2 billion.[4]

The Centers for Medicare & Medicaid Services (CMS)—the Department of Health and Human Services (HHS) agency responsible for administering the Medicare program and, in conjunction with the states, the Medicaid program—estimates Medicare and Medicaid FFS improper payments in part by reviewing provider medical record documentation to determine whether claims that providers submit for payment comply with program coverage policies. Among other types of improper payment errors, payments are improper when providers do not submit required documentation to support their claims, or the documentation submitted is insufficient to demonstrate compliance with coverage policies.[5] In fiscal

---

[2] See GAO, *High-Risk Series: Progress on Many High-Risk Areas, While Substantial Efforts Needed on Others*, GAO-17-317 (Washington, D.C.: February 2017). An improper payment is statutorily defined as any payment that should not have been made or that was made in an incorrect amount (including overpayments and underpayments) under statutory, contractual, administrative, or other legally applicable requirements. It includes any payment to an ineligible recipient, any payment for an ineligible service, any duplicate payment, payment for services not received (except where authorized by law), and any payment that does not account for credit for applicable discounts. 31 U.S.C. § 3321 note. Office of Management and Budget guidance provides that when an agency's review is unable to discern whether a payment was proper as a result of no or insufficient documentation, this payment must be considered an improper payment.

[3] Medicare and Medicaid also provide coverage through managed care, in which private managed care plans receive a periodic payment per beneficiary to provide a specific set of covered services to beneficiaries. In this report, we will focus solely on Medicare and Medicaid FFS improper payments.

[4] All Medicaid improper payment estimates in this report include federal and state spending.

[5] Medicaid tracks two types of improper payments due to insufficient documentation—one for payments when specific documentation is not provided, and another for payments for when the submitted documentation is insufficient. In this report we use the term insufficient documentation to refer to both types of improper payments.

year 2017, Medicare had an estimated $23.8 billion in improper payments due to providers submitting no or insufficient documentation, while Medicaid had an estimated $6.8 billion. CMS uses estimates of improper payments, including those due to no and insufficient documentation, to better understand the causes and extent of program risks, develop strategies to protect program integrity, and measure progress toward reducing improper payments.

We prepared this chapter under the authority of the Comptroller General to conduct evaluations to support congressional oversight of issues of national importance.[6] This chapter:

1) describes CMS's processes for obtaining and reviewing medical record documentation needed to estimate improper payments in Medicare and Medicaid FFS;
2) examines Medicare and Medicaid documentation requirements and factors that contribute to improper payments due to insufficient documentation; and
3) examines the extent to which reviews of medical record documentation provide state Medicaid agencies with actionable information on the underlying causes of improper payments.

To describe CMS's processes for obtaining and reviewing medical record documentation to estimate improper payments in Medicare and Medicaid FFS, we reviewed CMS documents for Medicare's Comprehensive Error Rate Testing (CERT) and Medicaid's Payment Error Rate Measurement (PERM) programs, respectively. CMS uses the CERT and PERM programs to identify improper payments and estimate Medicare and Medicaid improper payment amounts and rates. We interviewed CMS officials and CMS's CERT and PERM contractors regarding processes for obtaining and reviewing documentation, including steps taken by the contractors before determining that a claim is improper due to no or

---

[6] 31 U.S.C. § 717(b).

insufficient documentation.[7] We obtained data on the outreach to providers conducted by the CERT and PERM contractors to obtain documentation, and information on referrals of claims with evidence of potential fraud to other Medicare and Medicaid program integrity entities.

To examine Medicare and Medicaid documentation requirements and factors that contribute to improper payments due to insufficient documentation, we reviewed Medicare and Medicaid documentation requirements based on statutes, regulations, and other national and state coverage policies. We reviewed data on Medicare improper payment amounts for fiscal years 2005 through 2017; Medicaid improper payment amounts for fiscal years 2011 through 2017; and fiscal year 2017 estimated improper payment amounts and rates for four selected services types— home health, durable medical equipment (DME), laboratory, and hospice.[8] We selected these services based on their relatively high estimated amounts and rates of improper payments due to insufficient documentation, particularly in Medicare.[9] Specifically, these services accounted for $10.7 billion of $23.2 billion in Medicare improper payments due to insufficient documentation in fiscal year 2017.[10] We interviewed CMS officials; CERT and PERM contractor staff; officials from six state Medicaid agencies—California, Delaware, Indiana,

---

[7] The CERT and PERM programs each have two contractors—a statistical contractor that designs the programs' statistical sampling strategy and estimates improper payments, and a review contractor that reviews medical record documentation to determine whether claims were paid or denied properly. We interviewed the CERT and PERM statistical and review contractors.

[8] During the period of our review, fiscal year 2017 data represented the most recent, complete data for both Medicare and Medicaid FFS estimated improper payment amounts and rates. As of March 2019, CMS published the fiscal year 2018 Medicare FFS Supplemental Improper Payment Data report, but had not published the 2018 Medicaid FFS Supplemental Improper Payment Data report. See appendix II for fiscal year 2018 Medicare improper payment data.

[9] We examined documentation requirements and improper payments due to insufficient documentation for comparable services in both programs. Several Medicaid services with relatively high amounts and rates of insufficient documentation, such as personal support and outpatient prescription drug services, do not have comparable Medicare FFS services.

[10] The Medicare FFS category for estimated improper payments for laboratory services used in our analysis is specific to laboratories that are clinically independent and bill Medicare Part B, while the Medicaid estimated improper payments for laboratory services also includes X-ray and imaging services. While the categories are not directly comparable, we used the estimated improper payments to examine factors that contribute to improper payments for laboratory services due to insufficient documentation.

Massachusetts, Michigan, and New York; officials from provider associations representing the four selected services and an association representing physicians regarding the causes of improper payments due to insufficient documentation.[11] We selected the six states to review based on a range of estimated FFS improper payment rates, a range of FFS enrollment and expenditures, regional geographic diversity, and states representing each PERM cycle year.[12] The information we obtained from the six states and the provider associations cannot be generalized. We obtained illustrative examples from CMS of Medicare and Medicaid improper payments due to insufficient documentation for our selected services; these examples cannot be generalized. We also reviewed documentation about CMS initiatives to examine and revise provider documentation requirements. We assessed Medicare and Medicaid documentation requirements and processes for identifying improper payments due to insufficient documentation against Standards for Internal Control in the Federal Government.[13]

To examine the extent to which reviews of medical record documentation provide actionable information on the underlying causes of improper payments, we reviewed CMS's PERM and corrective action plan guidance, the PERM program's processes for estimating improper payments, national and state-level error rate data, and relevant statutes, regulations, and state coverage policies. We interviewed officials from the Office of Management and Budget (OMB) regarding agency requirements to estimate and address improper payments. We also interviewed officials from the six selected state Medicaid agencies regarding the PERM process, and reviewed the states' improper payments rates, causes of improper payments, and corrective action plans to address identified improper

---

[11] We interviewed officials from the following provider associations: American Association for Homecare, American Clinical Laboratory Association, American Medical Association, and National Association for Home Care & Hospice.

[12] The PERM computes an annual rolling average of improper payment rates across all states based on a 17-state, 3-year rotation cycle. For example, the fiscal year 2017 improper payment rate included states sampled as part of the 2015, 2016, and 2017 review years.

[13] See GAO, *Standards for Internal Control in the Federal Government*, GAO-14-704G (Washington, D.C.: Sept. 10, 2014). Internal control is a process effected by an entity's oversight body, management, and other personnel that provides reasonable assurance that the objectives of an entity will be achieved.

payments. The information we obtained from the six states cannot be generalized. Additionally, we reviewed guidance from the Association of Certified Fraud Examiners and interviewed officials from the HHS Office of the Inspector General (HHS-OIG) and the National Association of Medicaid Fraud Control Units to learn about best practices for investigative and review entities.[14] We assessed PERM processes and corrective actions plans against federal internal control standards and best practices for investigative and review entities.

The scope of our review is limited to the estimation of Medicare and Medicaid FFS improper payments and thus does not include other estimates of improper payments in these programs. In addition to the CERT's estimation of Medicare FFS improper payments, CMS has separate programs to estimate improper payments for Medicare's managed care and outpatient prescription drug programs, neither of which are included in the scope of our review. The PERM program estimates Medicaid improper payments for three key components of the Medicaid program—FFS, managed care, and beneficiary eligibility determinations. Our review only examines the FFS component of the PERM program, and within the FFS component, those improper payments identified through reviews of documentation. Medicaid FFS claims are also subject to data processing reviews and these reviews are not within the scope of our review.[15]

We conducted this performance audit from August 2017 to March 2019 in accordance with generally accepted government auditing standards. Those standards require that we plan and perform the audit to

---

[14] See Association of Certified Fraud Examiners, *Fraud Examiners Manual: 2018 International Edition* (Austin, Tex.: Association of Certified Fraud Examiners, 2018), 3.143- 3.144. The Association of Certified Fraud Examiners is an anti-fraud organization that provides anti-fraud training and education. The National Association of Medicaid Fraud Control Units is an organization that promotes interstate cooperation between Medicaid Fraud Control Units—state agencies that investigate Medicaid provider fraud, among other things.

[15] Medicaid data processing reviews examine claims to validate that states processed the claims correctly. The reviews identify improper payments that should not have been processed, such as payments to providers that did not comply with Medicaid enrollment and screening requirements. In recent years, data processing errors have accounted for the majority of Medicaid FFS improper payments. For example, data processing errors accounted for an estimated $35 billion in improper payments in fiscal year 2017.

obtain sufficient, appropriate evidence to provide a reasonable basis for our findings and conclusions based on our audit objectives. We believe that the evidence obtained provides a reasonable basis for our findings and conclusions based on our audit objectives.

BACKGROUND

Medicare and Medicaid FFS are federal health care programs, though there are certain distinctions between the programs' coverage and financing. Medicare coverage policies are generally established at the national level, and the program directly pays providers for services rendered. Medicaid is a federal-state program, and states are provided flexibility to design their coverage policies. State Medicaid agencies pay providers for services rendered, and the federal government and states share in the financing of the program, with the federal government matching most state expenditures.

Estimating Improper Payments in Medicare and Medicaid

The Improper Payments Information Act of 2002 (IPIA), as amended, requires federal executive branch agencies to report a statistically valid estimate of the annual amount of improper payments for programs identified as susceptible to significant improper payments.[16] To accomplish this, agencies follow guidance for estimating improper payments issued by OMB.[17] According to the HHS-OIG, which conducts annual compliance

---

[16] IPIA, Pub. L. No. 107-300, 116 Stat. 2350 (2002), as amended by the Improper Payments Elimination and Recovery Act of 2010, Pub. L. No. 111-204, 124 Stat. 2224, and the Improper Payments Elimination and Recovery Improvement Act of 2012, Pub. L. No. 112-248, 126 Stat. 2390 (2013), codified as amended at 31 U.S.C. § 3321 note. In lieu of reporting a statistically valid estimate, agencies may report an estimate that is otherwise appropriate, using an OMB-approved methodology.

[17] See Office of Management and Budget, *Appendix C to Circular No. A-123, Requirements for Effective Estimation and Remediation of Improper Payments*, OMB Memorandum M-15-02 (Washington, D.C.: October 2014). OMB updated its guidance in June 2018, effective

reviews and regularly reviews the estimation methodology for both the Medicare FFS and Medicaid improper payment measurement programs, the methodology for both programs' estimates comply with federal improper payment requirements.[18]

To estimate improper payments in Medicare and Medicaid FFS, respectively, CMS's CERT and PERM contractors randomly sample and manually review medical record documentation associated with FFS claims for payment from providers, also known as medical reviews.[19] The CERT and PERM programs project the improper payments identified in the sample to all FFS claims to estimate improper payment amounts and rates for the programs nationally for a given fiscal year. For Medicare, the CERT contractor conducted medical reviews on about 50,000 Medicare claims in fiscal year 2017. For Medicaid, the PERM contractor conducted medical reviews on nearly 31,000 Medicaid claims across fiscal years 2015, 2016, and 2017 to estimate fiscal year 2017 improper payments.[20] Although IPIA, as amended, only requires agencies to develop one improper payment estimate for each identified program, both the CERT and PERM programs also estimate national service-specific improper payment amounts and rates to identify services at high risk for improper payment. Additionally, the PERM program estimates state-level improper

---

starting in fiscal year 2018 unless otherwise noted in the revised guidance. See Office of Management and Budget, *Appendix C to Circular No. A-123, Requirements for Payment Integrity Improvement*, OMB Memorandum M-18-20 (Washington, D.C.: June 2018).

[18] The Improper Payments Elimination and Recovery Act of 2010 requires each agency's Office of Inspector General, including the HHS-OIG, to annually determine the compliance with the agency's improper payment requirements.

[19] Many improper payments can be identified only by manually reviewing documentation associated with claims to determine whether the claims met program coverage policies, such as medical necessity. Medical reviews are not conducted as part of normal processing of provider claims. For example, less than 1 percent of Medicare claims undergo such reviews.

[20] The PERM contractor conducted 7,599 medical reviews in fiscal year 2015, 9,964 medical reviews in fiscal year 2016, and 13,367 medical reviews in fiscal year 2017. In fiscal year 2017, the number of claims subject to medical review in a state was tied to that state's historical improper payment rates and payment variation. The number of claims subject to medical review per state ranged from 303 to 1,063. As a result, the total number of claims sampled nationally in a given year fluctuates based on the states reviewed that year. The PERM sampling methodology has since been updated under the final rule issued in 2017. See 82 Fed. Reg. 31,158 (July 5, 2017).

payment rates based on the amounts of improper payments identified through medical reviews in each state.[21]

The CERT and PERM contractors conduct medical reviews to determine whether claims were paid or denied properly in accordance with program coverage policies—including coverage policies based on statutes, regulations, other CMS coverage rules, and each state's coverage policies in the case of Medicaid.[22] To perform medical reviews, trained clinicians review documentation—such as progress notes, plans of care, certificates of medical necessity, and physician orders for services—to ensure that claims meet program coverage policies.

In general, Medicare and Medicaid documentation requirements define the documentation needed to ensure that services are medically necessary and demonstrate compliance with program coverage policies. For example, Medicare home health services must be supported by documentation demonstrating compliance with the coverage policy that beneficiaries be homebound, among other requirements.[23] Certain coverage policies and documentation requirements were implemented to help reduce the potential for fraud, waste, and abuse. For example, Medicare implemented a requirement that DME providers maintain documentation demonstrating proof of item delivery, to better ensure program integrity.[24] (Figure 1 presents an example of a progress note to support the medical necessity of Medicare home health services. See App. III for additional examples of provider documentation).

---

[21] The CERT program estimates improper payment rates for the geographic jurisdictions of Medicare Administrative Contractors, which process and pay claims, and perform program integrity activities in their jurisdictions.

[22] Other CMS coverage rules include Medicare national and local coverage determinations and coverage provisions in CMS interpretive manuals.

[23] To support homebound status, referring physician documentation must include clinical information documenting that beneficiaries meet certain criteria and generally detail the beneficiaries' inability to leave their home.

[24] See 65 Fed. Reg. 60,366 (Oct. 11, 2000) (codified at 42 C.F.R. § 424.57(c)(12)).

Progress Notes

Patient: Patient, John
DOB: 07/20/1943
Address: 321 Main St., Happyplace, MD 12345

Provider: Jane Doctor, M.D.
Date: 04/29/2018

Subjective:
CC:

1. Wound on left heel.

HPI:

Pt is here for evaluation of wound on left heel. Patient reports his daughter noticed the wound on patient's heel when washing his feet. Patient states he has difficulty with reaching his feet and his daughter will sometimes clean them for him. He reports he uses a shoe horn to put on his shoes.

ROS:

General: No weight change, no fever, no weakness, no fatigue.
Cardiology: No chest pain, no palpitations, no dizziness, no shortness of breath.
Skin: Wound on left lower heel, no pain.

Medical History: HTN, hyperlipidemia, hypothryroidism, DJD.
Medications: Zolpidem 10 mg tablet 1 tab once a day (at bedtime), Diovan HCl 12.5 mg-320 mg tablet 1 tab once a day, Lipitor 10 mg tablet 1 tab once a day.
Allergies: NKDA

Objective:
Vitals: Temp 96.8, BP 156/86, HR 81, RR 19, Wt 225, Ht 5'4"
Examination: General appearance pleasant. HEENT normal. Heart rate regular rate and rhythm, lungs clear, BS present, pulses 2+ bilaterally radial and pedal. Diminished pinprick sensation on bilateral lower extremities from toes to knees. Left heel wound measures 3 cm by 2 cm and 0.4 cm deep. Wound bed is red, without slough. Minimal amount of yellow drainage noted on removed bandage.

Assessment:
1. Open wound left heel

Plan:
1. **OPEN WOUND** Begin hydrocolloid with silver dressing changes. Minimal weight bear on left leg with a surgical boot on left foot. Begin home health for wound care, family teaching on wound care, and patient education on signs and symptoms of infection. The patient is now homebound due to minimal weight bearing on left foot and restrictions on walking to promote wound healing, he is currently using a wheelchair. Short-term nursing is needed for wound care, monitor for signs of infection, and education on wound care for family for dressing changes.

Follow Up: Return office visit in 2 weeks.

Jane Doctor, M.D. 4/29/2018

Provider: Jane Doctor, M.D.

Source: Centers for Medicare & Medicaid Services. | GAO-19-277.

Figure 1. Example Progress Note to Support Medicare Home Health Services.

The CERT and PERM contractors classify improper payments identified through medical review by the type of payment error. Two types of errors are related to documentation—no documentation and insufficient documentation.[25]

- **No documentation:** Improper payments in which providers fail to submit requested documentation or respond that they do not have the requested documentation.
- **Insufficient documentation:** Improper payments in which providers submit documentation that is insufficient to determine whether a claim was proper, such as when there is insufficient documentation to determine if services were medically necessary, or when a specific, required documentation element, such as a signature, is missing.

In fiscal year 2017, insufficient documentation comprised the majority of estimated FFS improper payments in both Medicare and Medicaid, with 64 percent of Medicare and 57 percent of Medicaid medical review improper payments. Improper payments stemming from insufficient documentation in Medicare FFS increased substantially starting in 2009, while insufficient documentation in Medicaid has remained relatively stable since 2011 (see Figure 2).[26]

CMS has attributed the increase in Medicare insufficient documentation since 2009 in part to changes made in CERT review criteria. Prior to 2009, CERT medical reviewers used "clinical inference" to determine that claims were proper even when specific documentation was missing if, based on other documentation and beneficiary claim histories, the reviewers could reasonably infer that the services were provided and medically necessary. Beginning with CMS's fiscal year 2009 CERT report, in response to 2008 HHS-OIG recommendations, CMS revised the criteria for CERT medical reviews to no longer allow clinical

---

[25] Other error types include improper payments due to incorrect procedure or service coding, and errors in which the service was determined to be not medically necessary based on program coverage policies.

[26] Prior to 2011, CMS did not separately report Medicaid improper payments for medical review error categories.

inference and the use of claim histories as a source of review information.[27] More recent policy changes that added to Medicare documentation requirements may have also contributed to the increase in insufficient documentation in Medicare FFS.

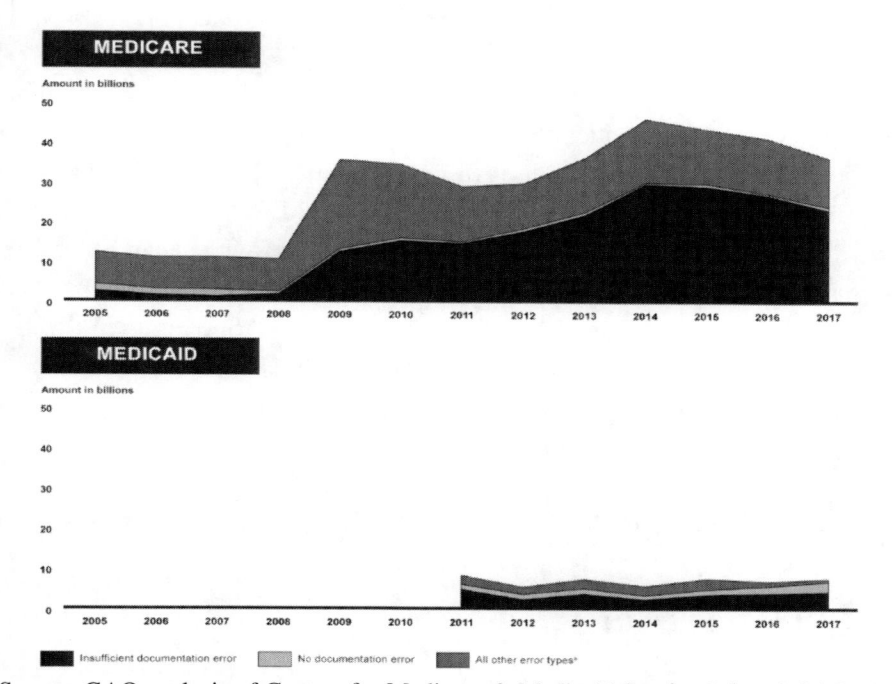

Source: GAO analysis of Centers for Medicare & Medicaid Services' data. | GAO-19-277.

Note: Prior to 2011, CMS did not separately report Medicaid improper payments for medical review error categories. Medical review refers to the process through which trained reviewers manually examine medical record documentation associated with provider claims to identify improper payments.

[a]All other error types include those not related to no or insufficient documentation, such as medical necessity, and incorrect coding errors.

Figure 2. Estimated Improper Payments Identified through Medical Review in Medicare and Medicaid Fee-for-service, Fiscal Years 2005-2017.

---

[27] HHS-OIG, *Medical Review of Claims for the Fiscal Year 2006 Comprehensive Error Rate Testing Program*, A-01-07-00508 (Washington D.C.: Aug. 2008). According to CMS and PERM contractor officials, PERM reviewers do not use clinical inference for Medicaid medical reviews.

CMS'S MEDICARE AND MEDICAID CONTRACTORS MAKE MULTIPLE ATTEMPTS TO CONTACT PROVIDERS TO OBTAIN DOCUMENTATION TO ESTIMATE IMPROPER PAYMENTS

Medicare's CERT and Medicaid's PERM contractors make multiple attempts to contact providers to request medical record documentation for medical reviews, and review all documentation until they must finalize the FFS improper payment estimate. The CERT and PERM contractors allow providers 75 days to submit documentation, though providers can generally submit late documentation up to the date each program must finalize its improper payment estimate, known as the cut-off date (See Figure 3). Both programs also contact providers to subsequently request additional documentation if the initial documentation submitted by the providers does not meet program requirements.

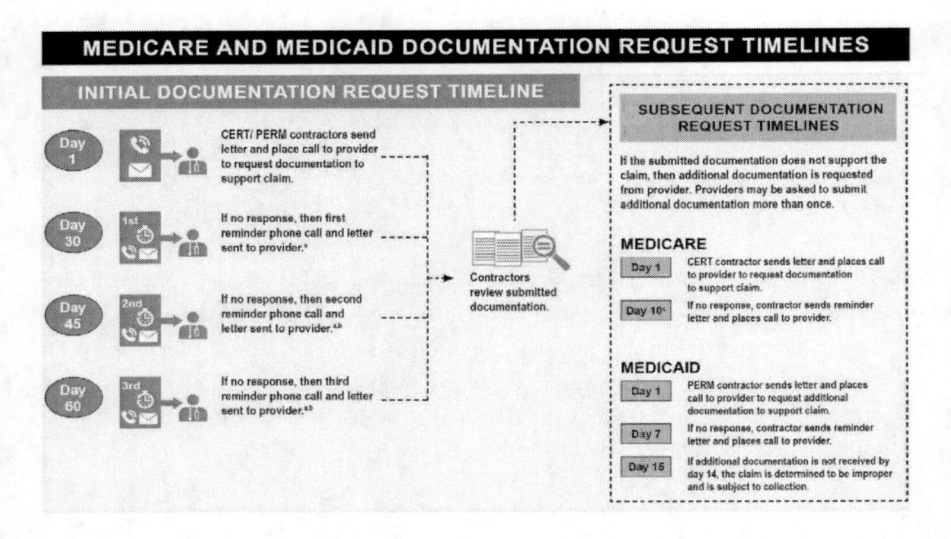

Figure 3. (Continued).

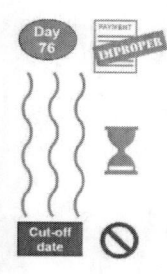

If documentation is not received by day 75, the claim is determined to be improper and is subject to collection.

Documents submitted late, up to the date each program must finalize its improper payment estimate, known as the cut-off date, are reviewed and improper payment estimates are adjusted based on the payment determination. Estimates are also adjusted based on claims that are successfully appealed prior to the cut-off date.

Source: GAO analysis of Centers for Medicare & Medicaid Services' documents. | GAO-19-277.

Note: Medicare's Comprehensive Error Rate Testing (CERT) and Medicaid's Payment Error Rate Measurement (PERM) contractors estimate Medicare's and Medicaid's improper payment rates.

[a]Reminder phone calls are placed around the time the letter is sent. For example, the CERT contractor places the first reminder call on day 25.

[b]Medicare providers are given 45 days to respond to the CERT contractor's documentation requests. However, providers are automatically given 15 day extensions on day 45 and day 60; claims are not determined to be improper until day 76.

[c]Unlike Medicaid, Medicare claims are not automatically determined to be improper after two weeks if additional documentation is not received. The CERT contractor told us that they may continue to contact providers to obtain additional documentation, though the claim will ultimately be determined to be improper if additional documentation is not provided.

Figure 3. Medicare and Medicaid Fee-for-Service Documentation Request Timelines to Estimate Improper Payments.

Initial Documentation Request

The CERT and PERM contractors make initial requests for documentation by sending a letter and calling the provider. After the initial provider request, if there is no response, the contractors contact the provider at least three additional times to remind them to submit the required documentation. If there is no response, the claim is determined to be improper due to no documentation. Claims are also classified as improper due to no documentation when the provider responds but cannot produce the documentation, such as providers that do not have the beneficiary's documentation or records for the date of service, among other reasons (see Table 1). For referred services, such as home health, DME, and laboratory services, the CERT contractor also conducts outreach to referring physicians to request documentation.[28]

Table 1. Medicare and Medicaid Estimated Fee-for-Service Improper Payments Due to No Documentation, by Cause, Fiscal Year 2017

Program	Cause	Number of improper payments due to no documentation	Total estimated improper payments (in millions of dollars)
Medicare Comprehensive Error Rate Testing (CERT)[a] program	No medical records were submitted (e.g., only cover sheet, billing records, etc.) or provider did not respond	112	Not available (NA)
	Provider said medical records not found for date of service or unable to locate records	49	NA
	Provider said beneficiary is not their patient	16	NA
	Provider no longer in business	4	NA
	Provider said that a third-party provider has medical record	3	NA
	Provider said that a different department within the provider fulfills documentation requests	2	NA
	CERT Total	186	613.2

---

[28] Certain nonphysician practitioners may refer for certain services. For example, nurse practitioners and physician assistants may refer for DME items. Additionally, institutional facilities refer for services, such as facilities that refer for home health services upon beneficiary discharge. For the purposes of this report, the term "referring physician" is inclusive of referring nonphysician practitioners and institutional facilities.

Program	Cause	Number of improper payments due to no documentation	Total estimated improper payments (in millions of dollars)
Medicaid Payment Error Rate Measurement (PERM) program	Provider did not respond to request	188	947.3
	Provider said services not provided on date requested	41	895.0
	Provider under fraud investigation[b]	27	85.7
	Provider said beneficiary not on file or in system	16	141.3
	Provider billed in error	12	112.3
	State could not locate provider	12	60.2
	Other[c]	32	244.1
	PERM Total	328	2,485.9

Source: GAO analysis of Centers for Medicare & Medicaid Services' (CMS) data. | GAO-19-277.

[a]The number of Medicare FFS improper payments may include the entire claim or a line-item within a claim for a service; a single claim or line-item within a claim may include multiple error causes. CMS does not project dollar amounts by cause for Medicare FFS because one claim or line-item could have more than one error cause.

[b]If a state notifies the PERM contractor that documentation for a specific provider is not available due to an ongoing investigation, the PERM stops requesting documentation from the provider, and the claim is cited as a no documentation error.

[c]Includes causes of no documentation errors with fewer than 10 improper payments, including instances where the provider said they could not locate the records; billed for the wrong beneficiary; are no longer in business; submitted documentation for the wrong date of service; or submitted only billing information.

For example, for a laboratory claim, the CERT contractor may contact the physician who ordered the laboratory test to request associated documentation, such as progress notes. Conversely, the PERM contractor told us they generally do not contact referring physicians to request documentation.

Subsequent Documentation Request

If a provider initially submits documentation that is insufficient to support a claim, then the CERT and PERM contractors subsequently request additional documentation.

- In fiscal year 2017, of the 50,000 claims in the CERT sample, the contractor requested additional documentation from 22,815 providers.[29] Providers did not submit additional documentation to sufficiently support 56 percent of the associated claims.
- For the 3 years that comprise the 2017 Medicaid improper payment rate, of the nearly 31,000 claims in the PERM sample, the contractor requested additional documentation for 5,448, and providers did not submit additional documentation to sufficiently support about 8 percent of the 5,448 claims.

In addition to having similar outreach to providers for obtaining documentation, the CERT and PERM contractors also have processes to refer suspected fraud to the appropriate program integrity entity, to ensure the accuracy of medical reviews, and to allow providers to dispute improper payment determinations.

Suspected Fraud

When CERT and PERM contractors identify claims with evidence of suspected fraud, they are required to refer the claims to other program integrity entities that are responsible for investigating suspected fraud.[30] CERT and PERM contractor officials said that in 2017, the CERT contractor referred 35 claims, and the PERM contractor did not make any referrals.

---

[29] Includes requests for documentation sent to both billing providers and referring physicians for the same claim. Accordingly, the number of claims subject to subsequent documentation requests is less than the number of providers.

[30] The CERT and PERM contractors do not estimate fraud in the programs, and their medical reviews are not intended or well-suited to detecting fraud. The CERT and PERM contractors review a random sample of claims and, according to CMS officials, generally only review a single claim for a given provider. Identifying suspected fraud requires activities specifically designed to detect the intent to defraud, such as identifying suspicious billing patterns of a particular provider.

Interrater Reliability (IRR) Reviews

As a part of their medical review processes, both the CERT and PERM contractors conduct IRR reviews, where two reviewers conduct medical reviews on the same claim and compare their medical review determinations. These IRR reviews ensure the consistency of medical review determinations and processes for resolving differences identified through the IRR reviews. CMS staff said that they also review a sample of the CERT and PERM contractors' payment determinations to ensure their accuracy.

- CERT: The contractor performs IRR reviews for at least 300 claims each month, including claims with and without improper payment determinations.
- PERM: The contractor conducts IRR reviews of all improper payment determinations, except improper payments due to no documentation, and 10 percent of all correctly paid claims in the sample, which combined was about 3,600 claims for the fiscal year 2017 national improper payment rate.[31]

Disputing Improper Payment Determinations

Both CERT and PERM contractors have processes in place for disputing the CERT or PERM contractor's improper payment determinations. These processes involve reviewing the claim, including any newly submitted documentation, and may result in upholding or overturning the initial improper payment determination. Improper payment determinations that are overturned prior to the CERT and PERM

---

[31] The PERM contractor does not conduct IRR reviews on improper payment determinations due to no documentation.

contractors' cut-off dates are no longer considered improper, and estimated improper payment amounts and rates are adjusted appropriately.[32]

- CERT: Medicare Administrative Contractors, which process and pay claims, may dispute the CERT contractor's improper payment determinations first with the CERT contractors and then, if desired, with CMS. Additionally, Medicare providers can appeal the CERT contractor's improper payment determinations through the Medicare appeals process.[33]
- PERM: State Medicaid officials may dispute the PERM contractor's improper payment determinations first with the PERM contractor and then, if desired, with CMS. Providers are not directly involved in this process; instead, providers can contact the state to appeal the improper payment determination.

DIFFERING MEDICARE AND MEDICAID DOCUMENTATION REQUIREMENTS MAY RESULT IN INCONSISTENT ASSESSMENTS OF PROGRAM RISKS

Differences in Documentation Requirements for Medicare and Medicaid May Result in Differing Improper Payment Rates and Assessments of Program Risks

We found that Medicare, relative to Medicaid, had a higher estimated FFS improper payment rate primarily due to insufficient documentation in fiscal year 2017. According to CMS data, across all services in fiscal year 2017, the rate of insufficient documentation was 6.1 percent for Medicare

---

[32] Because the PERM operates on a 3-year review cycle, improper payment determinations that are successfully overturned after the PERM cutoff date are not considered improper in subsequent year's improper payment estimates.

[33] For more information on Medicare's appeals process, see GAO, *Medicare Fee-for-Service: Opportunities Remain to Improve Appeals Process*, GAO-16-366 (Washington, D.C.: May 10, 2016).

and 1.3 percent in Medicaid, substantially greater than the difference in rates for all other types of errors, which were 3.4 and 1.0 percent, respectively. For home health, DME, and laboratory services, the insufficient documentation rate was at least 27 percentage points greater for Medicare than for Medicaid, and for hospice services, the rate was 9 percentage points greater (see Figure 4).

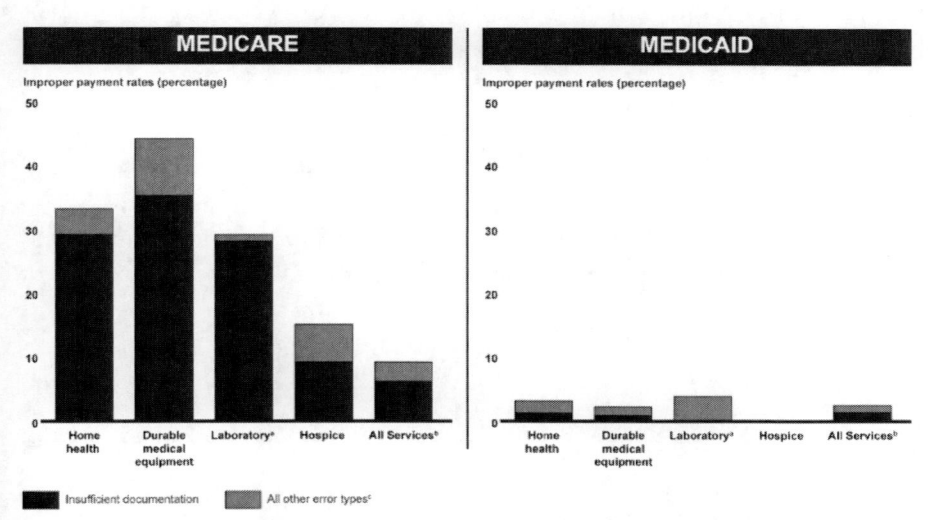

Source: GAO analysis of Centers for Medicare & Medicaid Services' data. | GAO-19-277.

Note: Medical review refers to the process through which trained reviewers manually examine medical record documentation associated with provider claims to identify improper payments.

[a]The Medicare laboratory service category is specific to laboratories that are clinically independent and bill Medicare Part B, while the Medicaid laboratory service category includes laboratory, X-ray, and imaging services. While the categories are not directly comparable, the magnitude of the differences in rates illustrates substantial differences in improper payments due to insufficient documentation for laboratory services.

[b]Totals are for all Medicare and Medicaid services, not only the services in the figure.

[c]All other error types include no documentation, medical necessity, incorrect coding, and other error categories.

Figure 4. Estimated Medical Review Improper Payment Rates in Medicare and Medicaid Fee-for-Service by Selected Service Categories, Fiscal Year 2017.

Differences between Medicare and Medicaid coverage policies and documentation requirements likely contributed to the substantial variation in the programs' insufficient documentation rates for the services we examined. Among the services we examined, there are four notable differences in coverage policy and documentation requirements that likely affected how the programs conducted medical reviews: face-to-face examinations; prior authorization; signature requirements; and documentation from referring physicians for referred services, as discussed below.

Examples of insufficient documentation in Medicare hospice

- Certification document did not include narrative information that sufficiently supported that the beneficiary had a life expectancy of less than 6 months.
- Certification document did not include the certification date span.

Centers for Medicare & Medicaid Services. | GAO-19-277.

Face-to-Face Examinations

In part to better ensure program integrity, the Patient Protection and Affordable Care Act established a requirement for referring physicians to conduct a face-to-face examination of beneficiaries as a condition of payment for certain Medicare and Medicaid services.[34] States were still in the process of implementing the policies for Medicaid in fiscal year 2017.

- Medicare requires home health and DME providers to submit documentation supporting that the referring physician conducted an examination when certifying the medical necessity of the

---

[34] CMS implemented face-to-face examination requirements for certain services based on provisions in the Patient Protection and Affordable Care Act. See Pub. L. No. 111-148, §§ 3132, 6407, 124 Stat.119, 430, 769 (2010) (codified as amended at 42 U.S.C. §§ 1395f, 1395f note, 1395n).

service. Hospice providers must submit documentation of a face-to-face examination when recertifying the medical necessity of hospice services for beneficiaries who receive care beyond 6 months after their date of admission.[35] (See sidebar for examples of insufficient documentation in Medicare hospice services.) CMS officials told us that documentation requirements for the face-to-face examination policy for home health services in particular led to an increase in insufficient documentation. When initially implemented in April 2011, home health providers had to submit separate documentation from the referring physician detailing the examination and the need for home health services. Beginning January 2015, CMS changed the requirement to allow home health providers to instead use documentation from the referring physician, such as progress notes, to support the examinations. CMS and several stakeholders attributed recent decreases in the home health improper payment rate to the amended documentation requirement (see Figure 5).

Examples of insufficient documentation in Medicaid

- Durable medical equipment provider did not submit physician order or proof of delivery for item.
- Plan of care submitted by home health agency did not apply to the sampled day of care associated with the claim.

Centers for Medicare & Medicaid Services. | GAO-19-277.

- CMS implemented a similar face-to-face examination policy for home health and DME services in Medicaid in 2016; however, the requirement likely did not apply to many claims subject to fiscal

---

[35] Medicare covers hospice services for beneficiaries with terminal illnesses who have been certified by a physician as having a life expectancy of 6 months or less, and recertified every 60 days for care beyond 6 months; each recertification must include a face-to-face examination. See 42 C.F.R. § 418.22(a)(4) (2017).

year 2017 PERM medical reviews.[36] Medicaid does not have a face-to-face policy for hospice services, and most states we interviewed did not have such policies. (See sidebar for examples of insufficient documentation in Medicaid.)

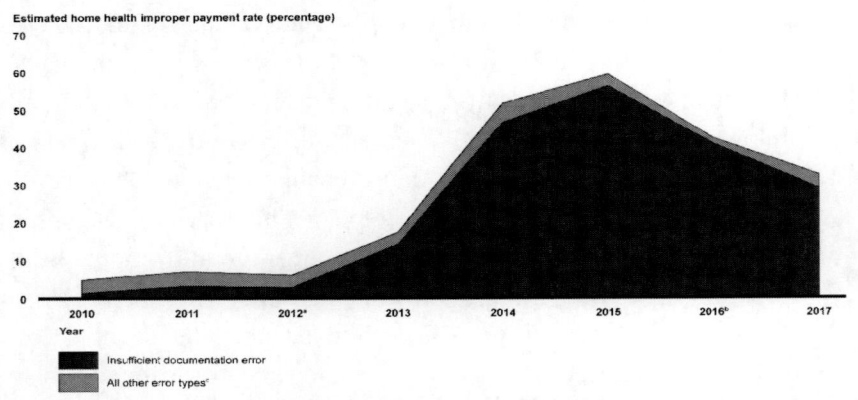

Source: GAO analysis of Centers for Medicare & Medicaid Services' data. | GAO-19-277.

[a]The Medicare sample for fiscal year 2012, which included claims from July 1, 2010 through June 30, 2011, was the first partial year in which claims subject to the documentation requirements associated with the face-to-face examination policy were reviewed.

[b]The Medicare sample for fiscal year 2016, which included claims from July 1, 2014 through June 30, 2015, was the first partial year in which claims subject to the amended documentation requirements were reviewed.

[c]All other error types include no documentation, medical necessity, incorrect coding, and other error categories.

Figure 5. Medicare Fee-for-Service Estimated Improper Payment Rate for Home Health Services, FY 2010-2017.

---

[36] In February 2016, CMS issued a final rule implementing the home health and DME requirement for Medicaid effective July 1, 2016. However, CMS delayed the compliance date for certain states for up to 2 years. See 81 Fed. Reg. 5530 (Feb. 2, 2016). Because of the requirements' delayed compliance date, Medicaid's 2017 improper payment estimate for home health and DME services likely did not include many claims subject to the face-to-face requirement.

Prior Authorization

Medicare does not have the same broad authority as state Medicaid agencies to implement prior authorization, which can be used to review documentation and verify the need for coverage prior to services being rendered. State Medicaid agencies we spoke with credit prior authorization with preventing improper payments from being paid in the first place.

- CMS has used prior authorization in Medicare for certain services through temporary demonstration projects and models, as well as one permanent program. In April 2018, we found that savings from a series of Medicare temporary demonstrations and models that began in 2012 could be as high as about $1.1 to $1.9 billion as of March 2017. We recommended that CMS take steps, based on its evaluations of the demonstrations, to continue prior authorization.[37]
- All six of our selected states use prior authorization in Medicaid for at least one of the four services we examined. In particular, all six selected states require prior authorization for DME, and five require prior authorization for home health.[38] Officials from several states noted that they often apply prior authorization to services at high risk for improper payments, and most told us that prior authorization screens potential improper payments before services are rendered. We did not evaluate the effectiveness of states' use of prior authorization, or review the documentation required by states for prior authorization. (See Figure 6 for an example state Medicaid prior authorization form.)

---

[37] See GAO, *Medicare: CMS Should Take Actions to Continue Prior Authorization Efforts to Reduce Spending*, GAO-18-341 (Apr 20, 2018). CMS neither agreed nor disagreed with our recommendation but said it would continue to evaluate the potential use of prior authorization in Medicare.

[38] These states may only subject certain services, such as specific DME items, to prior authorization.

1.1	Prior Authorization Request Form and Supplies

Prior Authorization Request Form – General Instructions

- Submit all requests 2 weeks prior to scheduled date of service.
- Incomplete forms will be returned and may delay the authorization process.
- Documentation related to the service(s) requested should be sent with the request.
- FAX or mail completed forms to the FAX number/address at right.

The Delaware Medical Assistance Program manuals are available for instructions and form downloads at https://medicaid.dhss.delaware.gov.

For questions, contact Provider Services at 800-999-3371.

Fax To: 1-302-255-4481

Department of Health & Social Services
Division of Medicaid & Medical Assistance
1901 N. Dupont Hwy, Lewis Building
P.O. Box 906
New Castle, DE 19720

Date Received: _____
FFS Eligibility Effective Date: _____

A. MEMBER INFORMATION

Name:	Member ID:	D.O.B.:
Address:		Phone:

Other Health Insurance (OHI) Information

Name of OHI:	Policy #:
Policyholder Name:	Policyholder SSN:

B. ORDERING PROVIDER INFORMATION

Name:	FAX #:
Address:	
Person Completing Form:	Telephone #:
NPI (National Provider ID) + Taxonomy:	

C. PRIMARY PHYSICIAN INFORMATION

Name:	FAX #:
NPI (National Provider ID) + Taxonomy:	Telephone #:

D. DME / HHC INFORMATION

Name:	Telephone #:
NPI (National Provider ID) + Taxonomy:	

E. SERVICE INFORMATION

Service Dates: FROM:	TO:	Continuation of Service ☐ Yes ☐ No

Diagnosis(es) / Service(s) / Procedure(s)

Diagnosis(es) / ICD-9 & ICD-10:				
CPT / HCPCS Codes:				

F. PLACE OF SERVICE:

	Out of State Provider: Yes ☐ No ☐
Name:	Telephone #:
NPI (National Provider ID) + Taxonomy:	FAX #:

CHECK SERVICES REQUESTED

☐ Durable Medical Equipment (DME)   ☐ Surgery / Diagnostic Testing / Other   ☐ Home Health Care (HHC) Service(s) – Please specify
☐ Private Duty Nursing   ☐ Skilled Nursing Visits   ☐ Home Health Aid (if greater than two hours per day)
☐ Physical Therapy   ☐ Occupational Therapy   ☐ Speech Therapy

Comments:

DO NOT WRITE BELOW THIS LINE

Date Received:	☐ Approved	☐ Denied	☐ Incomplete	Authorization #:
Comments:				

Signature:	Date:

Source: Delaware Department of Health and Social Services. | GAO-19-277.

Figure 6. Example State Medicaid Agency Prior Authorization Form.

Physician Signatures

While both Medicare and state Medicaid agencies require signatures on provider documents to ensure their validity, Medicare has detailed standards for what constitutes a valid signature.

- Medicare's signature standards address the validity of signatures in a variety of situations. For example, illegible signatures and initials on their own are generally invalid, though they are valid when over a printed name.[39]

Example of insufficient documentation in Medicare home health

- Documentation did not include actual clinical notes for the face-to-face encounter visit examination.

Example of insufficient documentation in Medicare durable medical equipment

- Documentation from the referring physician did not support the medical necessity for the specific type of catheter ordered.

Examples of insufficient documentation in Medicare laboratory

- Documentation from the referring physician did not support the order or an intent to order the billed laboratory tests.
- Documentation from the referring physician did not support that the beneficiary's currently has diabetes for a billed laboratory test for the management and control of diabetes.

Centers for Medicare & Medicaid Services. | GAO-19-277.

---

[39] For information on Medicare signature requirements, see CMS, Chapter 3, "Verifying Potential Errors and Taking Corrective Actions," *Medicare Program Integrity Manual*, accessed Nov. 2, 2018, https://www.cms.gov/Regulations-andGuidance/Guidance/Manuals/downloads/pim83c03.pdf.

- In Medicaid, PERM contractor staff told us that state agencies generally have not set detailed standards for valid signatures, and that reviewers generally rely on their judgment to assess signature validity.

Documentation for Referred Services

Medicare requires documentation from referring physicians to support the medical necessity of the referred services that we examined—home health, DME, and laboratory services—but Medicaid generally does not require such documentation.

- Medicare generally requires documentation from the referring physician, such as progress notes, to support the medical necessity of referred services.[40] CMS officials told us that Medicare requires such documentation from referring physicians to ensure that medical necessity determinations are independent of the financial incentive to provide the referred service, particularly as certain referred services are high risk for fraud, waste, and abuse.[41] (See sidebar for examples of insufficient documentation in Medicare home health, DME, and laboratory services.)
- In Medicaid, documentation requirements to support the medical necessity of referred services are primarily established by states, and states generally do not require documentation, such as progress notes from referring physicians, to support medical necessity. Further, PERM contractor staff told us that they

---

[40] Documentation generated by home health agencies, such as plans of care, can be used to support medical necessity in Medicare under certain conditions. See 42 U.S.C. § 1395f(a). Referring physicians must sign and incorporate the home health agencies' documentation into their medical records, and the home health agencies' documentation must be corroborated by the referring physicians' other medical records.

[41] We have previously reported on concerns related to improper payments in Medicare home health and DME services. See GAO, *Medicare: Improvements Needed to Address Improper Payments in Home Health*, GAO-09-185 (Washington, D.C.: Feb. 27, 2009) and GAO, *Medicare: CMS's Program Safeguards Did Not Deter Growth in Spending for Power Wheelchairs*, GAO-05-43 (Washington, D.C.: Nov. 17, 2004).

generally do not review such documentation when conducting medical reviews of claims for referred services.[42]

Officials from CMS, the CERT contractor, and provider associations told us that Medicare's documentation requirements for referred services present challenges for providers of referred services to submit sufficient documentation since they are dependent on referring physician documentation to support medical necessity. Some officials further stated that referring physicians may lack incentive to ensure the sufficiency of such documentation, as they do not experience financial repercussions when payments for referred services are determined to be improper. Officials told us that:

- It is generally not standard administrative practice for laboratories or DME providers to obtain referring physician documentation, and referring physicians may not submit them when the referred services are subject to medical review. For example, laboratories generally render services based solely on physician orders for specific tests, and generally do not obtain associated physician medical records.
- Referring physicians may not document their medical records in a way that meets Medicare documentation requirements to support the medical necessity of referred services. Officials from a physician organization told us that physicians refer beneficiaries for a broad array of services, and face challenges documenting their medical records to comply with Medicare documentation requirements for various referred services. We previously reported on CMS provider education efforts and recommended that CMS take steps to focus education on services at high risk for improper payments and to better educate referring physicians on

---

[42] The PERM contractor does not instruct providers of referred services to submit documentation, such as progress notes from referring physicians, to support medical necessity.

documentation requirements for DME and home health services.[43] CMS agreed with and has fully addressed our recommendation.

Medicare and Medicaid pay for many of the same services, to some of the same providers, and likely face many of the same underlying program risks.[44] However, because of differences in documentation requirements between the two programs, the same documentation for the same service can be sufficient in one program but not the other. The substantial variation in the programs' improper payment rates raise questions about how well their documentation requirements help in determining whether services comply with program coverage policies, and accordingly help identify causes of program risks. This is inconsistent with federal internal control standards, which require agencies to identify, analyze, and respond to program risks.[45]

CMS officials attributed any differences in the two programs' documentation requirements to the role played by the states in establishing such requirements under Medicaid, and told us that they have not assessed the implications of how differing requirements between the programs may lead to differing assessments of the programs' risks. CMS relies on improper payment estimates to help develop strategies to reduce improper payments, such as informing Medicare's use of routine medical reviews, educational outreach to providers, and efforts to address fraud.[46] Without a better understanding of how documentation requirements affect estimates of improper payments, CMS may not have the information it needs to

---

[43] See GAO, *Medicare Provider Education: Oversight of Efforts to Reduce Improper Billing Needs Improvement*, GAO-17-290 (Washington, D.C.: Mar 10, 2017).

[44] In recent years CMS has made efforts to align Medicare FFS and Medicaid program integrity efforts, indicating CMS's recognition of the overlaps and similarities of the risks faced by the two programs. For example, in 2010, CMS created the Center for Program Integrity, which consolidated the agency's program integrity functions for Medicare and Medicaid.

[45] See GAO-14-704G.

[46] CMS conducts routine medical reviews on Medicare claims as part of its strategy to reduce improper payments. For additional information on Medicare medical review efforts, see GAO, *Medicare: Claim Review Programs Could Be Improved with Additional Prepayment Reviews and Better Data*, GAO-16-394 (Washington, D.C.: Apr 13, 2016). For additional information on Medicare provider education, see GAO-17-290. For additional information on Medicare efforts to combat fraud, see GAO, *Medicare: CMS Fraud Prevention System Uses Claims Analysis to Address Fraud*, GAO-17-710 (Washington, D.C.: Aug 30, 2017).

effectively identify and analyze program risks, and develop strategies to protect the integrity of the Medicare and Medicaid programs.

CMS Has Ongoing Efforts to Examine Insufficient Documentation in Medicare and Revise Documentation Requirements

CMS's Patients over Paperwork initiative is an ongoing effort to simplify provider processes for complying with Medicare FFS requirements, including documentation requirements. Although CMS officials said this initiative is intended to help providers meet documentation requirements in both Medicare and Medicaid, current efforts only address Medicare documentation requirements. As part of the initiative, CMS solicited comments from stakeholders through proposed rulemaking on documentation requirements that often lead to insufficient documentation, and CMS officials stated that they have met with provider associations to obtain feedback. The initiative is generally focused on reviewing documentation requirements the agency has the authority to easily update, namely requirements that are based on CMS coverage rules, as opposed to requirements based on statute. Through this initiative, CMS has clarified and amended several Medicare documentation requirements. For example, CMS clarified Medicare documentation requirements for DME providers to support proof of item delivery.[47]

As part of another initiative to examine insufficient documentation in Medicare, CMS found that 3 percent of improper payments due to insufficient documentation were clerical in nature in fiscal year 2018.[48] For

---

[47] The documentation component of the Patients over Paperwork initiative is also known as the Documentation Requirements Simplification initiative. For a list of documentation requirements that have been updated, see https://www.cms.gov/Research-Statistics-Data-and-Systems/Monitoring-Programs/Medicare-FFS-Compliance-Programs/Simplifying Requirements.html (accessed December 21, 2018).

[48] For the purposes of our report, we refer to these errors as "clerical". CMS refers to these errors as "documentation non-compliance errors." For additional information on such errors, see *Department of Health and Human Services: FY2018 Agency Financial Report* (Washington, D.C., Nov. 14, 2018).

the CERT's fiscal year 2018 medical reviews, the CERT contractor classified whether improper payments due to insufficient documentation were clerical in nature—meaning the documentation supported that the service was covered and necessary, had been rendered, and was paid correctly, but did not comply with all Medicare documentation requirements. Such errors would not result in an improper payment determination if the documentation had been corrected. For example, such clerical errors may involve missing documentation elements that may be found elsewhere within the medical records.[49]

According to CMS officials, the information gathered on clerical errors may inform efforts to simplify documentation requirements. Specifically, CMS plans to use this information to help identify requirements that may not be needed to demonstrate medical necessity or compliance with coverage policies. CMS said that it does not plan to engage in similar efforts to examine insufficient documentation errors in Medicaid because of challenges associated with variations in state Medicaid documentation requirements and the additional burden it would place on states.

MEDICAID MEDICAL REVIEWS MAY NOT PROVIDE ACTIONABLE INFORMATION FOR STATES, AND OTHER PRACTICES MAY COMPROMISE FRAUD INVESTIGATIONS

Medicaid Medical Reviews Do Not Provide Robust State-Specific Information; Resulting Corrective Actions May Not Address the Most Prevalent Causes of Improper Payments

On a national basis, CMS's PERM program generates statistically valid improper payment estimates for the Medicaid FFS program. At the

---

[49] Claims for referred services that were determined to be improper because of issues with referring physician medical record documentation were not considered clerical errors because such payments do not sufficiently document the medical necessity of the referred services.

state level, however, CMS officials told us that the PERM contractor's medical reviews do not generate statistically generalizable information about improper payments by service type and, as a result, they do not provide robust state-specific information on the corrective actions needed to address the underlying causes of improper payments.

Table 2. Number of Improper Medicaid Fee-for-Service Payments Identified through the Payment Error Rate Measurement (PERM) Program's Medical Reviews, Fiscal Year 2017

Number of Improper Payments Identified through Medical Reviews[a]	Number of States in Range	Amount of Improper Payments[b] (dollars)	Percent of Improper Payments[c]
1-10	27	97,491	7
11-25	10	141,201	10
26-40	6	476,261	34
41-55	5	431,630	31
56-67	3	255,791	18
Total 918	51	1,402,374	100

Source: GAO analysis of Centers for Medicare & Medicaid Services' data. | GAO-19-277.

Note: Table includes data from all 50 states and the District of Columbia.

[a]Medical review refers to the process through which trained reviewers manually examine medical record documentation associated with provider claims to identify improper payments. The total presented includes 40 medical technical deficiencies that do not result in an improper payment, such as an incorrect date of service that is less than 7 calendar days before or after the actual date of service.

[b]Amount of improper payments is the aggregated total dollars identified through medical reviews of a sample of claims. It is not the projected amount of improper payments in Medicaid fee-for-service.

[c]Percent of improper payments represents the percent of the sample subjected to medical reviews. It is not the percent of all improper payments in Medicaid fee-for-service.

According to CMS, the number of improper payments identified through medical reviews is too small to generate robust state-specific results. In fiscal year 2017, the PERM contractor identified 918 improper payments nationwide out of nearly 31,000 claims subjected to medical reviews.[50] More than half of all states had 10 or fewer improper payments identified through medical reviews in fiscal year 2017, and these made up about 7 percent of total sample improper payments identified through medical reviews (see Table 2).

According to CMS officials, estimating improper payments for specific service types within each state with the same precision as the national estimate would involve substantially expanding the number of medical reviews conducted and commensurately increasing PERM program costs. CMS officials also estimated federal spending on PERM Medicaid FFS medical reviews at about $8 million each year, which does not include state costs, the federal share of the state costs, or providers' costs.[51] Of our six selected states, officials from one state said that data on service-specific improper payment rates at the state level would be useful, though officials had reservations about increasing sample sizes because of the resources involved in doing so.[52]

CMS requires state Medicaid agencies to develop corrective actions to rectify each improper payment identified. However, since the Medicaid review sample in a state typically is not large enough to be statistically generalizable by service type, the identified improper payments may not be representative of the prevalence of improper payments associated with different services within the state. Accordingly, corrective actions designed to rectify specific individual improper payments may not address the most prevalent underlying causes of improper payments. For example, state Medicaid officials in four of our six states said that most improper payments identified through PERM medical reviews are unique one-time events. Federal internal control standards require agencies to identify and analyze program risks so they can effectively respond to such risks, and OMB expects agencies to implement corrective actions that address

---

[50] This total includes 40 medical technical deficiencies which do not result in an improper payment, such as an incorrect date of service that is less than 7 calendar days before or after the actual date of service.

[51] CMS estimates that the PERM medical reviews cost providers $93,192 annually.

[52] None of the six states we spoke with formally tracked their state's spending on PERM medical reviews.

underlying causes of improper payments.[53] Without estimates that provide information on the most prevalent underlying causes of improper payments within a state, particularly by service type, a state Medicaid agency may not be able to develop appropriate corrective actions or prioritize activities to effectively address program risks. Corrective actions that do not address the underlying causes of improper payments are unlikely to be an effective use of state resources.

Increasing sample sizes of the PERM is one approach that could improve the usefulness of the medical reviews for states—but other options also exist. For example, PERM findings could be augmented with data from other sources—such as findings from other CMS program integrity efforts, state auditors, and HHS-OIG reports. States conduct their own program integrity efforts, including medical reviews, to identify improper payments and state Medicaid officials we spoke with in four of our six selected states said that they largely rely on such efforts to identify program risks. One state's Medicaid officials said that state-led audits allow them to more effectively identify—and subsequently monitor—services that are at risk for improper payments in the state. CMS also could use data from other sources on state-specific program risks to help design states' PERM samples.[54] These options could help CMS and the states better identify the most prevalent causes of improper payments and more effectively focus corrective actions and program integrity strategies to address program risks.[55]

---

[53] See GAO-14-704G.

[54] Several state and federal entities are responsible for identifying and addressing improper payments in Medicaid. For example, state Medicaid agencies typically have designated entities responsible for ensuring Medicaid program integrity, and states are generally required to establish Medicaid Fraud Control Units. In addition, state auditors are responsible for assessing financial management and accountability in state government agencies and programs. On the federal level, CMS provides states with guidance related to statutory and regulatory requirements, technical assistance, and education about program integrity best practices, and HHS-OIG helps oversee Medicaid program integrity through its audits, investigations, and program evaluations.

[55] We previously recommended that CMS take steps to mitigate risks in Medicaid managed care that are not measured in the PERM. CMS agreed with this recommendation but has not yet taken steps to address it. See GAO, *Medicaid: CMS Should Take Steps to Mitigate Program Risks in Managed Care*, GAO-18-291 (Washington, D.C.: May 7, 2018).

CMS Policy May Limit State Identification of Medicaid Providers under Fraud Investigation

State Medicaid agencies may, but are not required to, determine whether providers included in the PERM sample are under fraud investigation and notify the PERM contractor. Under CMS policy, when a state notifies the PERM contractor of a provider under investigation, the contractor will end all contact with the provider to avoid compromising the fraud investigation, and the claim will be determined to be improper, due to no documentation.[56] In fiscal year 2017, of the 328 Medicaid improper payments due to no documentation, 27 (8 percent) from five states, according to CMS, were because the provider was under fraud investigation.

If a state Medicaid agency does not notify the PERM contractor about providers under fraud investigation, the PERM contractor will conduct its medical review, which involves contacting the provider to obtain documentation as a part of its normal process, and communicate about improper payment determinations. Contacting providers that are under fraud investigation as part of PERM reviews could interfere with an ongoing investigation, such as in the following ways we identified based on information from the Association of Certified Fraud Examiners and others.

- The contact by the PERM contractor to request documentation, although unrelated to the fraud investigation, may give the impression that the provider is under heightened scrutiny. This could prompt the provider to change its behavior, or to destroy, falsify, or create evidence. These actions could in turn disrupt or complicate law enforcement efforts to build a criminal or civil case.
- The PERM contractor's communication about improper payment determinations may prompt states to conduct educational outreach

---

[56] This is similar to Medicare, where claims that are not reviewed because the provider is under fraud investigation, are also considered improper due to no documentation.

to the provider about proper billing procedures. This may inadvertently change the billing practices of a fraudulent provider for whom law enforcement is trying to establish a pattern of behavior.

We found that states may not have processes to determine whether providers included in the PERM sample are under fraud investigation. Of the six states we spoke with, officials from two states said they did not have a mechanism in place to identify providers under fraud investigation. However, it is a best practice for investigative and review entities to communicate and coordinate with one another to determine if multiple entities are reviewing the same provider and for investigators to work discreetly without disrupting the normal course of business, based on our analysis of information from the Association of Certified Fraud Examiners and others. Accordingly, investigators should be aware of other government entities that are in contact with providers under investigation, such as the PERM contractor, who may contact providers multiple times to request documentation, and refer identified improper payments for recovery. If multiple entities are reviewing the same provider, one entity may be directed to pause or cease its activities, such as a PERM medical review, to reduce the risk of compromising an active fraud investigation. CMS has stated that it is not the agency's intention to negatively impact states' provider fraud investigations and, therefore, it has provided states the option to notify the PERM contractor of any providers under investigation to avoid compromising investigations.[57] However, CMS does not require states to determine whether providers under PERM medical

---

[57] CMS also stated that the agency does not believe that PERM reviews will compromise investigations because requests for medical records are routine and should be expected by providers participating in Medicaid. The agency also noted that it is not necessarily the case that the claims selected for PERM review are the subject of the ongoing investigation. See 72 Fed. Reg. 50,490, 50,495 (Aug. 31, 2007); 75 Fed. Reg. 48,816, 48,821 (Aug. 11, 2010). Officials from the National Association of Medicaid Fraud Control Units noted that medical reviews are an expected part of Medicaid participation and that contacting providers may have limited impact on fraud investigations. However, they also said that some providers under fraud investigation may be sensitive to any contact by reviewers and may change their behaviors in response.

reviews are also under fraud investigation, which creates the potential that PERM reviews could interfere with ongoing investigations.

State Medicaid agencies may not have incentives to notify the PERM contractor of providers under fraud investigation, as doing so will automatically result in a no documentation error, which increases states' improper payment rates. Medicaid officials from one state we spoke with said that while they check whether providers subject to PERM reviews are under investigation for fraud, they do not report these instances to the PERM contractor because the PERM contractor would find a no documentation error and the claim would be cited as improper, increasing the state's improper payment rate. Officials from another state said this policy penalizes states, in the form of higher state-level improper payment rates that may reflect poorly on states. Additionally, officials from this state were reluctant to develop corrective actions for improper payments stemming from such no documentation errors.

CONCLUSION

CMS and states need information about the underlying causes of improper payments to develop corrective actions that will effectively prevent or reduce future improper payments in Medicare and Medicaid FFS. The substantial variation in Medicare and Medicaid estimated improper payment rates for the services we examined raise questions about how well the programs' documentation requirements ensure that services were rendered in accordance with program coverage policies. While our study focused on certain services with high rates of insufficient documentation, differences in documentation requirements between the programs may apply to other services as well. Without examining how the programs' differing documentation requirements affect their improper payment rates, CMS's ability to better identify and address FFS program risks and design strategies to assist providers with meeting requirements may be hindered.

At the state level, PERM medical reviews do not provide robust information to individual states. CMS's requirements to address individual improper payments may lead states to take corrective actions that may not fully address underlying causes of improper payments identified through medical review, and may misdirect state efforts to reduce improper payments. Absent a more comprehensive review of existing sources of information on the underlying causes of Medicaid improper payments, CMS and states are missing an opportunity to improve their ability to address program risks. In addition, the lack of a requirement for state Medicaid agencies to determine whether providers whose claims are selected for PERM medical reviews are also under fraud investigation risks compromising ongoing investigations. Further, citing such claims as improper payments in states' estimated improper payment rates may discourage state Medicaid agencies from notifying the PERM contractor that a provider is under investigation.

RECOMMENDATIONS

We are making the following four recommendations to CMS:

- The Administrator of CMS should institute a process to routinely assess, and take steps to ensure, as appropriate, that Medicare and Medicaid documentation requirements are necessary and effective at demonstrating compliance with coverage policies while appropriately addressing program risks. (Recommendation 1)
- The Administrator of CMS should take steps to ensure that Medicaid medical reviews provide robust information about and result in corrective actions that effectively address the underlying causes of improper payments. Such steps could include adjusting the sampling approach to reflect state-specific program risks, and working with state Medicaid agencies to leverage other sources of information, such as state auditor and HHS-OIG findings. (Recommendation 2)

- The Administrator of CMS should take steps to minimize the potential for PERM medical reviews to compromise fraud investigations, such as by directing states to determine whether providers selected for PERM medical reviews are also under fraud investigation and to assess whether such reviews could compromise investigations. (Recommendation 3)
- The Administrator of CMS should address disincentives for state Medicaid agencies to notify the PERM contractor of providers under fraud investigation. This could include educating state officials about the benefits of reporting providers under fraud investigation, and taking actions such as revising how claims from providers under fraud investigation are accounted for in state-specific FFS improper payment rates, or the need for corrective actions in such cases. (Recommendation 4)

AGENCY COMMENTS AND OUR EVALUATION

We provided a draft of this chapter to HHS for comment, and its comments are reprinted in appendix I. HHS also provided us with technical comments, which we incorporated in the report as appropriate.

HHS concurred with our first recommendation that CMS institute a process to routinely assess and ensure that Medicare and Medicaid documentation requirements are necessary and effective. HHS stated that CMS's Patients over Paperwork initiative is focused on simplifying Medicare documentation requirements and noted that for the Medicaid program, CMS will identify and share documentation best practices with state Medicaid agencies. CMS's Patients over Paperwork initiative may help CMS streamline Medicare documentation requirements. However, we believe CMS should take steps to assess documentation requirements in both programs to better understand the variation in the programs' requirements and their effect on estimated improper payment rates. Without an assessment of how the programs' documentation requirements affect estimates of improper payments, CMS may not have the information it needs to ensure that Medicare and Medicaid documentation requirements are effective at demonstrating compliance and appropriately address program risks.

HHS did not concur with our second recommendation that CMS ensure that Medicaid medical reviews provide robust information about and result in corrective actions that effectively address the underlying causes of improper payments. HHS noted that increasing the PERM sample size would involve increasing costs and state Medicaid agencies' burden, and that incorporating other sources of information into the PERM sample design could jeopardize the sample's statistical validity. HHS also commented that it already uses a variety of sources to identify and take corrective actions to address underlying causes of improper Medicaid payments. We acknowledge that increasing the sample size would increase the costs of the PERM medical review program, though the level of improper payments warrants continued action. Further, under the current approach, we found that CMS and state Medicaid agencies are expending time and resources developing and implementing corrective actions that may not be representative of the underlying causes of improper payments in their states. It is important that corrective actions effectively and efficiently address the most prevalent causes of improper payments, and our report presents options that could improve the usefulness of the PERM's medical reviews—such as augmenting medical reviews with other sources of information during the development of corrective actions. We continue to believe that corrective actions based on more robust information would help CMS and state Medicaid agencies more effectively address Medicaid program risks.

HHS concurred with our third and fourth recommendations that CMS minimize the potential for PERM medical reviews to compromise fraud investigations and address disincentives for state Medicaid agencies to notify the PERM contractor of providers under fraud investigation. In its comments HHS described the actions it has taken and is considering taking to implement these recommendations.

We are sending copies of this chapter to appropriate congressional committees, to the Secretary of Health and Human Services, the Administrator of CMS, and other interested parties.

James Cosgrove
Director, Health Care

Carolyn L. Yocom
Director, Health Care

List of Addressees

The Honorable Charles E. Grassley
Chair

The Honorable Ron Wyden
Ranking Member
Committee on Finance
United States Senate

The Honorable Richard Neal
Chair

The Honorable Kevin Brady
Ranking Member
Committee on Ways and Means
House of Representatives

The Honorable Devin Nunes
Ranking Member
Committee on Ways and Means
Subcommittee on Health
House of Representatives

The Honorable Mike Kelly
Ranking Member
Committee on Ways and Means
Subcommittee on Oversight
House of Representatives

APPENDIX I: COMMENTS FROM THE DEPARTMENT OF HEALTH AND HUMAN SERVICES

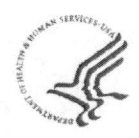

DEPARTMENT OF HEALTH & HUMAN SERVICES   OFFICE OF THE SECRETARY

Assistant Secretary for Legislation
Washington, DC 20201

MAR 0 8 2019

Carolyn Yocom
Director, Health Care
U.S. Government Accountability Office
441 G Street NW
Washington, DC 20548

Dear Ms. Yocom:

Attached are comments on the U.S. Government Accountability Office's (GAO) report entitled, *"Medicare and Medicaid: CMS Should Assess Documentation Necessary to Identify Improper Payments"* (GAO-19-277).

The Department appreciates the opportunity to review this report prior to publication.

Sincerely,

Matthew D. Bassett
Assistant Secretary for Legislation

Attachment

GENERAL COMMENTS OF THE DEPARTMENT OF HEALTH AND HUMAN SERVICES (HHS) ON THE GOVERNMENT ACCOUNTABILITY OFFICE'S DRAFT REPORT ENTITLED: MEDICARE AND MEDICAID: CMS SHOULD ASSESS DOCUMENTATION NECESSARY TO IDENTIFY IMPROPER PAYMENTS (GAO-19-277)

The Department of Health and Human Services (HHS) appreciates the opportunity to review and comment on this draft report. HHS is strongly committed to program integrity efforts in the Medicare and Medicaid programs.

As part of its program integrity efforts, HHS uses the Comprehensive Error Rate Testing (CERT) and Payment Error Rate Measurement (PERM) programs to estimate the Medicare Fee-For-Service (FFS) and Medicaid improper payment rates, respectively. It is important to note the improper payment rates are not "fraud rates" but simply a measurement of payments made (including both underpayments and overpayments) that did not meet statutory, regulatory, or administrative requirements. Both the CERT and PERM programs include reviews of medical records to determine whether claims were paid or denied properly in accordance with Federal and, in the case of Medicaid, state requirements. These reviews can be time-consuming for HHS, states, and providers; involve documentation requirements that can be complex and for which the source of legal authority may be distributed among multiple statutes, regulations, and subregulatory guidance and manuals; and often require several interactions with the provider to make sure required documentation has been provided.

As part of HHS' initiative to put patients first and reduce unnecessary provider burden in the Medicare FFS program, in 2017 HHS launched the Patients over Paperwork Initiative. This initiative includes the evaluation of potential ways to streamline regulations and other policies with the goals of reducing unnecessary burden, increasing efficiencies, and improving the beneficiary experience. As part of Patients over Paperwork, HHS implemented the Documentation Requirements Simplification Initiative, which is a process to simplify documentation requirements and eliminate any that are no longer needed. As part of this initiative, HHS is inviting feedback from providers and other stakeholders; reviewing current regulatory requirements and sub-regulatory guidance; analyzing medical review findings, such as findings from the Targeted Probe and Educate program; and undertaking conversations with internal stakeholders. Through this initiative, HHS has already clarified and amended several Medicare documentation requirements.[1]

HHS is also developing a Provider Documentation Manual, which will eventually list all of the documentation required for Medicare payment in one central location. The purpose of the Provider Documentation Manual is to reduce the need for providers and suppliers to reference multiple HHS documents by providing checklists that providers or suppliers can use to ensure their documentation is complete. The Provider Documentation Manual does not replace policy and coverage manuals and does not create any new requirements. HHS is posting draft sections of the manual on our website and accepting comments on these.[2]

---

[1] https://www.cms.gov/Research-Statistics-Data-and-Systems/Monitoring-Programs/Medicare-FFS-Compliance-Programs/SimplifyingRequirements.html

[2] https://www.cms.gov/Research-Statistics-Data-and-Systems/Monitoring-Programs/Medicare-FFS-Compliance-Programs/ReducingProviderBurden.html

GENERAL COMMENTS OF THE DEPARTMENT OF HEALTH AND HUMAN SERVICES (HHS) ON THE GOVERNMENT ACCOUNTABILITY OFFICE'S DRAFT REPORT ENTITLED: MEDICARE AND MEDICAID: CMS SHOULD ASSESS DOCUMENTATION NECESSARY TO IDENTIFY IMPROPER PAYMENTS (GAO-19-277)

For the Medicaid program, a state generally establishes documentation requirements in regulations and other guidance documents, based on its coverage policies and an individualized determination of what requirements are appropriate in that state. As the Government Accountability Office (GAO) notes in its report, the Medicaid program is a federal-state partnership that allows states the flexibility to establish and effectively manage their Medicaid programs, along with HHS oversight to ensure that federal statutory and regulatory requirements are met. Because documentation requirements can differ based on the structure of a Medicaid program and each state's determination of appropriate policy, HHS believes the states are better suited than the Federal Government to establish such documentation requirements. Lastly, requiring a state to revise its documentation requirements could also impose a significant burden on both the state and Medicaid providers.

HHS already uses a variety of sources that can help to identify the root causes of improper payments and target corrective actions to reduce improper payments. These sources include, but are not limited to, CERT, PERM, and Medicaid Eligibility Quality Control program results; Corrective Action Plans that are developed from improper payment measurement data; data analysis performed on Medicare and Medicaid claims; state program integrity reviews and site visits; and feedback from stakeholders, including state Medicaid agencies, GAO, and the HHS Office of Inspector General (OIG).

In recent years, these efforts have led to a reduction in the Medicare FFS and Medicaid improper payment rates. The 2018 Medicare FFS improper payment rate is 8.12 percent, which is the lowest such rate since 2010. The 2018 Medicaid improper payment rate is 9.79 percent; it has fallen since 2016, when it was 10.48 percent. HHS continues to explore additional opportunities to reduce the improper payment rates.

We remain committed to collaborating across HHS and with stakeholders to address potential vulnerabilities, strengthen our program integrity efforts, and minimize unnecessary administrative burden for our partners.

GAO's recommendations and HHS' responses are below.

GAO Recommendation
The Administrator of CMS should institute a process to routinely assess, and take steps to ensure, as appropriate, that Medicare and Medicaid documentation requirements are necessary and effective at demonstrating compliance with coverage policies while appropriately addressing program risks.

HHS Response
HHS concurs with GAO's recommendation.

In fact, as GAO notes in its report, HHS has already established this process. As mentioned above, the Documentation Requirements Simplification Initiative aims to simplify documentation requirements and eliminate requirements that are no longer needed. Through this initiative, HHS has already clarified and amended several Medicare documentation requirements.

GENERAL COMMENTS OF THE DEPARTMENT OF HEALTH AND HUMAN SERVICES (HHS) ON THE GOVERNMENT ACCOUNTABILITY OFFICE'S DRAFT REPORT ENTITLED: MEDICARE AND MEDICAID: CMS SHOULD ASSESS DOCUMENTATION NECESSARY TO IDENTIFY IMPROPER PAYMENTS (GAO-19-277)

HHS concurs with GAO's recommendation for Medicaid. Medicaid is a federal-state partnership, and states generally establish documentation requirements in regulations and other guidance documents based on coverage policies and an individualized determination of what requirements are appropriate in that state. CMS will work to identify best practices for documentation requirements and share those with states.

GAO Recommendation

The Administrator of CMS should take steps to ensure that Medicaid medical reviews provide robust information about and result in corrective actions that effectively address the underlying causes of improper payments. Such steps could include adjusting the sampling approach to reflect state-specific program risks, and working with state Medicaid agencies to leverage other sources of information, such as state auditor and HHS-OIG findings.

HHS Response

HHS does not concur with this recommendation.

As stated above, HHS uses a variety of sources to identify the root causes of improper payments and target corrective actions to reduce improper payments. HHS can encourage states to utilize findings from all sources when developing corrective actions to address identified root causes of improper payments. However, using data from other sources, such as state auditor and OIG findings, on state-specific program risks to adjust the PERM sampling approach could jeopardize the statistical validity of the PERM program.

Under the PERM program in FY 2017, HHS subjected nearly 31,000 Medicaid FFS claims to medical reviews at a cost of nearly $8 million. Those costs did not include state costs, the federal share of state costs, or provider costs. As GAO notes in its report, estimating improper payments for specific service types within states with the same precision as the national estimate would require substantially expanding the number of medical reviews conducted and lead to an increase in PERM costs and burden on states and providers.

GAO Recommendation

The Administrator of CMS should take steps to minimize the potential for PERM medical reviews to compromise fraud investigations, such as by directing states to determine whether providers selected for PERM medical reviews are also under fraud investigation and to assess whether such reviews could compromise investigations.

HHS Response

HHS concurs with GAO's recommendation.

Regarding current policy, HHS already provides guidance in the January 2018 PERM Manual to states to determine whether providers included in the PERM sample are under fraud investigation.[3] Should states determine that PERM medical reviews could compromise an investigation, they may

---

[3] https://www.cms.gov/Research-Statistics-Data-and-Systems/Monitoring-Programs/Medicaid-and-CHIP-Compliance/PERM/Downloads/FY17PERMManual.pdf

notify the PERM contractor and the contractor will end all contact with the provider. HHS will consider clarifying our policy to help ensure that such providers are not contacted in the first instance.

HHS will explore additional actions it can take to minimize the potential for PERM medical reviews to compromise fraud investigations.

GAO Recommendation

The Administrator of CMS should address disincentives for state Medicaid agencies to notify the PERM contractor of providers under fraud investigation. This could include educating state officials about the benefits of reporting providers under fraud investigation, and taking actions such as revising how payments from providers under fraud investigation are accounted for in state-specific FFS improper payment rates, or the need for corrective actions in such cases.

HHS Response

HHS concurs with this recommendation.

HHS will consider actions to minimize the negative impact on states of reporting providers under fraud investigation, such as increasing education to states about the minimal impact of any associated PERM errors and eliminating the requirement to develop corrective actions to address these errors.

HHS thanks GAO for their efforts on this issue and looks forward to working with GAO on this and other issues in the future.

APPENDIX II: FISCAL YEAR 2018 MEDICARE IMPROPER PAYMENT DATA

During the period of our review, fiscal year 2017 data represented the most recent, complete data for both Medicare and Medicaid fee-for-service (FFS) estimated improper payment amounts and rates. As of March 2019, the Centers for Medicare & Medicaid Services published the fiscal year 2018 Medicare FFS Supplemental Improper Payment Data report, but had not published the 2018 Medicaid FFS Supplemental Improper Payment Data report. The Centers for Medicare & Medicaid Services estimated Medicare FFS spending of $389 billion, and $32 billion in improper payments.

Table 3 below presents updated fiscal year 2018 data for the Medicare improper payment data by the services examined in our report.

Table 3. Medicare Fee-for-Service Estimated Improper Payment Amounts and Rates by Selected Service Categories, Fiscal Year 2018

Service	Improper payments (dollars in billions)	Improper payment rate (percentage)	Improper payments due to insufficient documentation (dollars in billions)	Insufficient documentation improper payment rate (percentage)[a]	Improper payments due to all other error types (dollars in billions)[b]	All other error types improper payment rate (percentage)[c]
Home health	3.2	17.6	2.0	10.9	1.2	6.7
Durable medical equipment	2.6	35.5	2.0	27.7	.6	7.8
Laboratory[d]	1.0	28.2	.9	25.8	.1	2.4
Hospice	2.1	11.7	1.2	7.0	.8	4.6
All services[e]	31.6	8.1	18.3	4.7	13.3	3.4

Source: GAO analysis of Centers for Medicare & Medicaid Services' data. | GAO-19-277.

Note: Totals may not sum due to rounding.

[a]The rate at which all payments for the service were improper because of insufficient documentation errors.

[b]All other error types includes no documentation, medical necessity, incorrect coding, and other error categories.

[c]The rate at which all payments for the service were improper because of all other error types, which includes no documentation, medical necessity, incorrect coding, and other error categories.

[d]The Medicare laboratory service category is specific to laboratories that are clinically independent and bill Medicare Part B.

[e]Total for all Medicare services, not just services in the table.

APPENDIX III: SELECTED EXAMPLES OF MEDICAL RECORD TEMPLATES FOR MEDICARE AND MEDICAID PROVIDERS

Medicare and state Medicaid agencies have released template medical record documentation, such as certificates of medical necessity and plans of care that providers may use to document information necessary to ensure compliance with coverage policies. This appendix presents examples of such templates.

Figure 7 presents a Medicare template that referring physicians can use to certify beneficiary need for home health services.

DRAFT

Use of this template is voluntary / optional

Home Health Plan of Care / Certification

Patient information

Last name: _____ First name: _____ MI: ___

DOB (MM/DD/YYYY): _____ Gender: ___ M ___ F ___ Other Medicare ID: _____

F2F evaluation information

Date of F2F visit (MM/DD/YYYY): _____

Other relevant information

Patient HI Claim No: _____ Medical Record Number: _____

Initial start of care date (MM/DD/YYYY): _____

For recertification: start/end of this episode of care (MM/DD/YYYY): _____ / _____

Advanced Directives: _____ Yes _____ No   *If yes, describe:* _____

Pertinent diagnoses (status: acute, chronic, acute-chronic, resolved, resolving, managed)

ICD-10-CM	Description	Start date	Status

Relevant procedures (e.g. surgical) (include code from ICD-10-PCS, HCPCS, CPT when available)

Code	Description	Date Performed

Home Health Services Plan of Care / Certification Template Draft R2.0 7/9/2018   Page 1 of 1

Source: Centers for Medicare & Medicaid Services. | GAO-19-277   Part 1 of 6

Figure 7. (Continued).

DRAFT

Pertinent medications (Status: N=New, A=Active, C=Changed, D=Discontinued) (include RxNorm if known)

RxNorm	Description	Dose	Frequency	Route	Status
___	___	___	___	___	___
___	___	___	___	___	___
___	___	___	___	___	___
___	___	___	___	___	___
___	___	___	___	___	___
___	___	___	___	___	___
___	___	___	___	___	___
___	___	___	___	___	___
___	___	___	___	___	___

Allergies (all) (include RxNorm for medication allergies when known)

RxNorm	Description	RxNorm	Description
___	___	___	___
___	___	___	___

Functional assessment:

Functional limitations (check all that apply): ___ Amputation, ___ Bowel/bladder (Incontinence), ___ Contracture, ___ Hearing, ___ Paralysis, ___ Endurance, ___ Speech, ___ Legally blind, ___ Dyspnea with minimal exertion, ___ Angina with minimal exertion or at rest, ___ CVA/hemiparalysis/paralysis/dysphonia, ___ Confined to wheelchair, ___ Fall risk

Other functional limitations: _____

Activities permitted (check all that apply): ___ Complete bedrest, ___ Bedrest BRP, ___ Up as tolerated, ___ Transfer bed/chair, ___ Partial weight bearing, ___ Independent at home, ___ Crutches, ___ Cane, ___ Wheelchair, ___ Walker, ___ No restrictions

Other activities permitted: _____

Mental status (check all that apply) ___ Oriented, ___ Comatose, ___ Forgetful, ___ Depressed, ___ Disoriented, ___ Lethargic, ___ Agitated

Other mental, psychosocial, and cognitive status observations: _____

Home Health Services Plan of Care / Certification Template Draft R2.0 7/9/2018   Page **2** of **6**

Figure 7. (Continued).

DRAFT

DME and supplies: _____

Safety measures: _____

Nutritional requirements: _____

Prognosis: ___ Poor, ____ Guarded, ___ Fair, ____ Good, ___ Excellent

Additional clarification: _____

Description of risk for emergency department visits and hospital readmission and all necessary interventions to address risk: _____

Patient and caregiver education and training to facilitate timely discharge: _____

Patient-specific interventions and education: measurable outcomes, goals and status identified by the HHA and patient. Status: Proposed, Accepted, Planned, In Progress, On Target, Ahead of Target, Behind Target, Sustaining, Achieved, On Hold, Cancelled, Rejected

Intervention/Education	Measurable Outcomes /Goals	Status

Home Health Services Plan of Care / Certification Template Draft R2.0 7/9/2018   Page **3** of **6**

Figure 7. (Continued).

DRAFT

Orders (may be satisfied with an attached, signed order template)

Intermittent skilled nursing services (*complete all that are required*)

Administration of medications	Frequency:_____	Duration:_____
Tube feeding	Frequency:_____	Duration:_____
Wound care	Frequency:_____	Duration:_____
Catheters	Frequency:_____	Duration:_____
Ostomy care	Frequency:_____	Duration:_____
NG and tracheostomy aspiration/care	Frequency:_____	Duration:_____
Psychiatric evaluation and therapy	Frequency:_____	Duration:_____
Teaching/training	Frequency:_____	Duration:_____
Observe/assess	Frequency:_____	Duration:_____
Complex care plan management	Frequency:_____	Duration:_____
Rehabilitation nursing	Frequency:_____	Duration:_____
Other: _____	Frequency:_____	Duration:_____
Other: _____	Frequency:_____	Duration:_____

Justification and signature if the patient's sole skilled service need is for skilled oversight of unskilled services (management and evaluation of the care plan or complex care plan management):

_____

_____

_____ Physician's Signature: _____

Therapy services (*complete all that are required*)

Physical therapy

Restore patient function	_____	
Perform maintenance therapy	_____	
Therapeutic exercises	Frequency:_____	Duration:_____
Gait and balance training	Frequency:_____	Duration:_____
ADL training	Frequency:_____	Duration:_____
Other: _____	Frequency:_____	Duration:_____

Occupational therapy

Restore patient function	_____	
Perform maintenance therapy	_____	
Therapeutic exercises	Frequency:_____	Duration:_____
ADL training	Frequency:_____	Duration:_____
Other: _____	Frequency:_____	Duration:_____

Home Health Services Plan of Care / Certification Template Draft R2.0 7/9/2018   Page **4** of **6**

Figure 7. (Continued).

DRAFT

Speech-language pathology

Restore language function	_____	
Restore cognitive function	_____	
Swallowing	Frequency:_____	Duration:_____
Perform maintenance therapy	Frequency:_____	Duration:_____
Other: _____	Frequency:_____	Duration:_____

Other Services

Home health aide services	Frequency:_____	Duration:_____
Medical social services	Frequency:_____	Duration:_____

Verbal Orders

Date/time	Order	Taken by
_____	_____	_____
_____	_____	_____
_____	_____	_____
_____	_____	_____

Frequency, Duration and Purpose of Visits:

Frequency	Duration	Purpose
_____	_____	_____
_____	_____	_____
_____	_____	_____

Additional Items from the HHA and/or physician: _____

Rehabilitation potential

Service/Intervention	Rehabilitation potential
_____	_____
_____	_____
_____	_____

Home Health Services Plan of Care / Certification Template Draft R2.0 7/9/2018   Page 5 of 6

Figure 7. (Continued).

DRAFT

Discharge plans _____

_____

_____

_____

Communicated to primary care physician:

Provider name _____ *Date:* _____ *By:* _____

Preparer signature: _____

Last name: _____ First name: _____ MI: ___ Suffix: _____

Date (MM/DD/YYYY): _____

Signature, Name, Date and NPI of physician signing the POC/Certification:

If this is a subsequent episode:

How much longer will skilled services be needed? _____

I certify that this patient is confined to his/her home (as outlined in section 30.1.1 in Chapter 7 of the Medicare Benefit Policy Manual (Pub. 100-02)) and needs intermittent skilled nursing care, physical therapy and/or speech therapy or continues to need occupational therapy. The patient is under my care, and I have authorized services on this plan of care and will periodically review the plan. The patient had a face-to-face encounter with an allowed provider type and the encounter was related to the primary reason for home health care.

I authenticate that the verbal orders recorded above are accurate.

Signature: _____

Last name: _____ First name: _____ MI: ___ Suffix: _____

Date (MM/DD/YYYY): _____ NPI: _____

Date physician signed POC was received by the HHA (MM/DD/YYYY): _____

Revisions of the POC communicated to:

Role	Name	Date	By
Patient/Caregiver			
Certifying Provider			
Ordering Provider			
Ordering Provider			
Ordering Provider			

Home Health Services Plan of Care / Certification Template Draft R2.0 7/9/2018   Page 6 of 6

Figure 7. Medicare Home Health Services Certification Draft Template.

Figure 8 presents a Medicare template that referring physicians can use to certify beneficiary need for home oxygen supplies.

DEPARTMENT OF HEALTH AND HUMAN SERVICES
CENTERS FOR MEDICARE & MEDICAID SERVICES

Form Approved OMB
No. 0938-0679
Expires 02/2020

CERTIFICATE OF MEDICAL NECESSITY CMS-484 OXYGEN

DME 484.03

SECTION A: Certification Type/Date: INITIAL ___/___/___ REVISED ___/___/___ RECERTIFICATION ___/___/___

PATIENT NAME, ADDRESS, TELEPHONE and MEDICARE ID	SUPPLIER NAME, ADDRESS, TELEPHONE and NSC or NPI #
(___) ___ - ___ Medicare ID	(___) ___ - ___ NSC or NPI #
PLACE OF SERVICE _____ Supply Item/Service Procedure Code(s):	PT DOB ___/___/___ Sex ___ (M/F) Ht. ___ (in) Wt ___
NAME and ADDRESS of FACILITY if applicable (see reverse)	PHYSICIAN NAME, ADDRESS, TELEPHONE and UPIN or NPI #
	(___) ___ - ___ UPIN or NPI #

SECTION B: Information in this Section May Not Be Completed by the Supplier of the Items/Supplies.

EST. LENGTH OF NEED (# OF MONTHS): _____ 1–99 (99=LIFETIME) | DIAGNOSIS CODES: _____

ANSWERS	ANSWER QUESTIONS 1–9. (Check Y for Yes, N for No, or D for Does Not Apply, unless otherwise noted.)
a) _____ mm Hg b) _____ % c) ___/___/___	1. Enter the result of recent test taken on or before the certification date listed in Section A. Enter (a) arterial blood gas PO2 and/or (b) oxygen saturation test; (c) date of test.
❏1 ❏2 ❏3	2. Was the test in Question 1 performed (1) with the patient in a chronic stable state as an outpatient, (2) within two days prior to discharge from an inpatient facility to home, or (3) under other circumstances?
❏1 ❏2 ❏3	3. Check the one number for the condition of the test in Question 1: (1) At Rest; (2) During Exercise; (3) During Sleep
❏Y ❏N ❏D	4. If you are ordering portable oxygen, is the patient mobile within the home? If you are not ordering portable oxygen, check D.
_____ LPM	5. Enter the highest oxygen flow rate ordered for this patient in liters per minute. If less than 1 LPM, enter an "X".
a) _____ mm Hg b) _____ % c) ___/___/___	6. If greater than 4 LPM is prescribed, enter results of recent test taken on 4 LPM. This may be an (a) arterial blood gas PO2 and/or (b) oxygen saturation test with patient in a chronic stable state. Enter date of test (c).
	ANSWER QUESTIONS 7-9 ONLY IF PO2 = 56–59 OR OXYGEN SATURATION = 89 IN QUESTION 1
❏Y ❏N	7. Does the patient have dependent edema due to congestive heart failure?
❏Y ❏N	8. Does the patient have cor pulmonale or pulmonary hypertension documented by P pulmonale on an EKG or by an echocardiogram, gated blood pool scan or direct pulmonary artery pressure measurement.
❏Y ❏N	9. Does the patient have a hematocrit greater than 56%?

NAME OF PERSON ANSWERING SECTION B QUESTIONS, IF OTHER THAN PHYSICIAN (Please Print):
NAME_____ TITLE_____ EMPLOYER_____

SECTION C: Narrative Description of Equipment and Cost

(1) Narrative description of all items, accessories and option ordered; (2) Suppliers charge; and (3) Medicare Fee Schedule Allowance for each item, accessory, and option (see instructions on back)

SECTION D: PHYSICIAN Attestation and Signature/Date

I certify that I am the treating physician identified in Section A of this form. I have received Sections A, B and C of the Certificate of Medical Necessity (including charges for items ordered). Any statement on my letterhead attached hereto, has been reviewed and signed by me. I certify that the medical necessity information in Section B is true, accurate and complete, to the best of my knowledge, and I understand that any falsification, omission, or concealment of material fact in that section may subject me to civil or criminal liability.

PHYSICIAN'S SIGNATURE_____ DATE ___/___/___
Signature and Date Stamps Are Not Acceptable.

Form CMS-484 (02/17)

Source: Centers for Medicare & Medicaid Services. | GAO-19-277

Figure 8. Medicare Certificate of Medical Necessity Template for Oxygen Supplies.

Figure 9 presents a template from the Indiana Medicaid program that hospices may use to document beneficiary plans of care.

MEDICAID HOSPICE PLAN OF CARE			
State Form 48731 (R3 / 2-09) / OMPP 0011		The information contained on this completed form is **CONFIDENTIAL** according to 405 IAC 1-16, 5-2-19.1, 5-2-10.2, 5-5-1, and 5-34.	**Reset Form**

A. RECIPIENT INFORMATION

Primary hospice diagnosis (ICD-#)

Name of recipient (last, first, middle initial)

Recipient's Medicaid number

Recipient's Social Security number

B. HOSPICE PROVIDER INFORMATION

Name of hospice provider

Hospice provider number

C. ASSESSMENT: Complete the following using the problem severity code listed at the bottom of the chart.

ASSESSMENT	PROBLEM SEVERITY CODE	ASSESSMENT	PROBLEM SEVERITY CODE
Altered Physical Comfort		Altered Urinary Elimination	
Altered Respiratory Status		Altered Bowel Elimination	
Altered Cardiovascular Status		Altered Sleep Pattern	
Altered Nutritional Status		Altered Grief/Spiritual (patient)	
Altered Skin Integrity		Altered Grief/Spiritual (family)	
Altered Mobility Status		Altered Oral Mucosa	
ACTIVITIES OF DAILY LIVING	**PROBLEM SEVERITY CODE**	**ACTIVITIES OF DAILY LIVING**	**PROBLEM SEVERITY CODE**
Eating / Feeding		Toileting	
Grooming / Hygiene		Continence	
Bathing		Transferring	
Dressing		Mobility	

PROBLEM SEVERITY CODE

0 = None: no problem present
1 = Problem: controlled at time of assessment
2 = Mild: function could be improved.

3 = Moderate: able to function with support
4 = Marked: able to function only with daily intervention
5 = Severe: incapacitated by the problem

D. SERVICES: Document the proposed services for this benefit period (*include frequency and expected outcome*).

Services Required	Frequency	Expected Outlook
Skilled Nursing		

(*Continued on the reverse side*)

Source: Indiana Family and Social Services Administration. | GAO-19-277   Part 1 of 2

Figure 9. (Continued).

E. SERVICES (continued)		
Services Required	Frequency	Expected Outlook
Home Health		
Therapy		
DME		
Pharmacy		
Spiritual		
Other enhanced services		

F. SIGNATURES: Date and sign the following. Signatures must represent the Medical Director as well as two signatures from any of the other disciplines listed above.		
Signature	Title	Date (month, day, year)
Signature	Title	Date (month, day, year)
Signature	Title	Date (month, day, year)

Source: Indiana Family and Social Services Administration. | GAO-19-277   Part 2 of 2

Figure 9: Indiana Hospice Plan of Care Template.

In: Government Reports on Health Care …   ISBN: 978-1-53615-844-1
Editor: Eric Beyer   © 2019 Nova Science Publishers, Inc.

Chapter 5

PRIVATE HEALTH INSURANCE: ENROLLMENT REMAINS CONCENTRATED AMONG FEW ISSUERS, INCLUDING IN EXCHANGES[*]

United States Government Accountability Office

ABBREVIATIONS

CMS	Centers for Medicare & Medicaid Services
CO-OP	Consumer Operated and Oriented Plan
HHS	Department of Health and Human Services
PPACA	Patient Protection and Affordable Care Act
SHOP	Small Business Health Options Program

---

[*] This is an edited, reformatted and augmented version of United States Government Accountability Office; Report to Congressional Committees; Accessible Version, Publication No. GAO-19-306, dated March 2019.

WHY GAO DID THIS STUDY

A highly concentrated health insurance market may indicate less competition and could affect consumers' choice of issuers and the premiums they pay. In 2014, PPACA required the establishment of health insurance exchanges—a new type of marketplace where individuals and small groups can compare and select among insurance plans sold by participating issuers—and the introduction of other reforms that could affect market concentration and competition among issuers. GAO previously reported that enrollment through these newly established exchanges was also generally concentrated.

PPACA included a provision for GAO to study market concentration. This chapter describes changes in the concentration of enrollment among issuers in (1) overall individual, small group, and large group markets, and (2) individual and small group exchanges.

GAO determined market share in the overall markets using enrollment data from 2015 and 2016 that issuers are required to report annually to the Centers for Medicare & Medicaid Services (CMS) and compared that data to 2011 through 2014 enrollment data GAO analyzed in previous reports. GAO determined market share in the exchanges from 2015 through 2017 using other sources of enrollment data from CMS and states. For all data sets, GAO used the most recent data available.

WHAT GAO FOUND

Enrollment in private health insurance plans continued to be concentrated among a small number of issuers in 2015 and 2016. In the overall large group market (coverage offered by large employers), small group market (coverage offered by small employers), and individual market (coverage sold directly to individuals), the three largest issuers held 80 percent of the market or more in at least 37 of 51 states. This is similar to what GAO previously reported for 2011 through 2014.

GAO also found that within the overall individual and small group markets in each state, the health insurance exchanges established by the Patient Protection and Affordable Care Act (PPACA) were also concentrated from 2015 to 2017.

- For the individual market exchanges, in each year, three or fewer issuers held 80 percent or more of the market, on average, in at least 46 of the 49 state exchanges for which GAO had data. Further, the largest issuers increased their market share in about two-thirds of exchanges. The number of issuers participating in a market and their market shares can affect concentration, and many individual exchanges generally had a decreasing number of participating issuers over time.
- For the small group market exchanges, in each year, three or fewer issuers held 80 percent or more of the market in at least 42 of the 46 state exchanges for which GAO had data. The small group exchanges also had slight changes in issuer participation and market share over this time period.

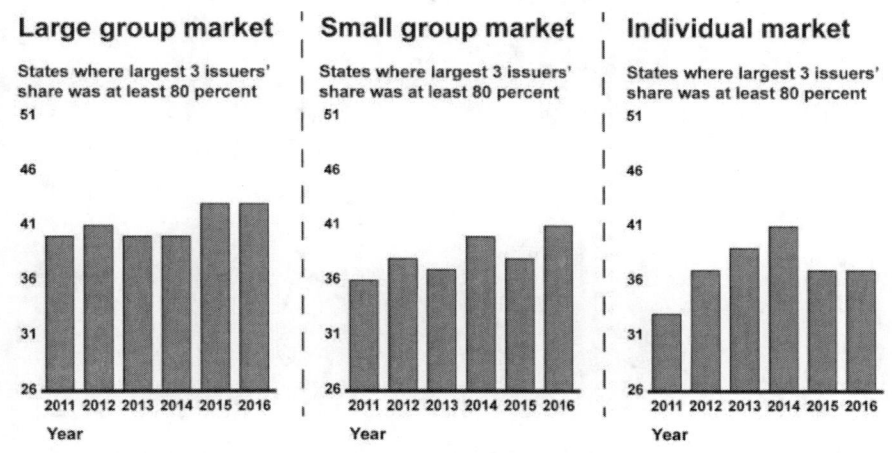

Source: GAO analysis of data from the Centers for Medicare & Medicaid Services. | GAO-19-306.

Number of States Where the Three Largest Issuers Had at Least 80 Percent of Enrollment, by Market, 2011-2016.

GAO received technical comments on a draft of this chapter from the Department of Health and Human Services and incorporated them as appropriate.

March 21, 2019
Congressional Committees

Historically, the market for health insurance sold by private issuers has been highly concentrated—that is, a small number of issuers in the market enrolled most of the people in that market.[1] We previously reported that, from 2010 through 2013, enrollment in most states was concentrated among the largest issuers in each of the three types of health insurance markets: the large group market (coverage offered by large employers), the small group market (coverage offered by small employers), and the individual market (consisting mainly of coverage sold directly to individual consumers who lack access to group coverage).[2] We also reported that these trends continued in 2014, which was the first year in which a number of provisions from the Patient Protection and Affordable Care Act (PPACA) took effect.[3] For example, we found that enrollment was similarly concentrated among a small number of issuers during the first year of operation of the health insurance exchanges that were created under PPACA. Health insurance exchanges are markets that operate within each state's overall individual and small group market where eligible individuals and small employers can compare and select among qualified

---

[1] We use the term "issuer" when referring to the entities that are licensed by a state to engage in the business of insurance in that specific state.

[2] GAO, *Private Health Insurance: Concentration of Enrollees among Individual, Small Group, and Large Group Insurers from 2010 through 2013*, GAO-15-101R (Washington, D.C.: Dec. 1, 2014).
Federal law defines a small employer as having an average of 1 to 50 employees during the preceding calendar year; however, states may apply this definition based on an average of 1 to 100 employees. See 42 U.S.C. §§ 300gg-91(e)(4), 18024(b)(2).

[3] GAO, *Private Health Insurance: In Most States and New Exchanges Enrollees Continued to be Concentrated among Few Issuers in 2014*, GAO-16-724 (Washington, D.C.: Sept. 6, 2016). See Pub. L. No. 111-148, 124 Stat. 119 (2010) (hereafter, "PPACA"), as amended by the Health Care and Education Reconciliation Act of 2010, Pub. L. No. 111-152, 124 Stat. 1029 (2010). In this report, references to PPACA include any amendments made by the Health Care and Education Reconciliation Act of 2010.

insurance plans offered by participating issuers.[4] A highly concentrated insurance market may indicate less competition and could affect consumers' choice of issuers and the premiums they pay.

PPACA also included a provision for us to conduct a study on competition and concentration in health insurance markets.[5] For the current study, we describe changes in the concentration of enrollment among issuers in each state's:

1) overall individual health insurance market, including the individual market exchange;
2) overall small group health insurance market, including the small group exchange; and
3) overall large group health insurance market.

To analyze changes in concentration in the overall individual, small group, and large group markets in each state, we analyzed 2015 and 2016 Medical Loss Ratio data that PPACA requires issuers to report annually to the Department of Health and Human Services' (HHS) Centers for Medicare & Medicaid Services (CMS).[6] Data for 2016 were the most recently available at the time of our analysis. We previously analyzed 2011 through 2014 data from this same source in our prior reports on concentration; we present that information alongside our new analyses in this chapter.[7] Within the overall individual, small group, and large group markets for each of the 51 states, we determined the state-level market

---

[4] States may establish separate individual and small group exchanges or a single exchange to serve both individuals and small groups. In this report, the term "state" includes the District of Columbia.

[5] PPACA, § 1322(i), 124 Stat. at 192. PPACA directs us to report to Congress biennially beginning in 2014. See GAO-15-101R and GAO-16-724 for our prior work in response to this mandate.

[6] PPACA required that all issuers report Medical Loss Ratio data to CMS, which include the percent of premiums the issuers spent on their enrollees' medical claims and quality initiatives, known as their medical loss ratio. These data also include enrollment data that can be used to calculate the market share for fully insured health plans. We did not examine self-funded health plans, where small and large employers set aside funds to pay for employee health care rather than pay premiums to an issuer to do so. The data include state-level enrollment data and are publicly available on the CMS website.

[7] GAO-16-724.

share for each issuer by calculating the ratio of the total number of covered life-years for each issuer in a state to the total number of covered life-years in that state.[8]

To analyze changes in concentration in the individual market exchanges, we obtained data from CMS and states for 2015, 2016, and 2017, the most recently available at the time of our analyses.[9] CMS operated individual market exchanges—referred to as federally facilitated exchanges—in about three-quarters of states.[10] For these states, CMS provided us with data from its data warehouse, the Multidimensional Insurance Data Analytics System, for each enrollee who obtained health insurance coverage through federally facilitated exchanges for 2015, 2016, or 2017.[11] These data included, among other information, the enrollees' coverage start and end dates, the issuers from which the enrollees purchased coverage, and the states and rating areas— geographic areas established by states and used, in part, by issuers to set premium rates—in which the enrollees lived.[12] For the remaining states, which operated their own individual market exchanges, each state generally provided us with

---

[8] One way to measure beneficiary enrollment is by calculating covered life-years, which measure the average number of lives insured, including dependents, during the reporting year. Rather than a point in time measurement, this measure accounts for changes in enrollment that occur throughout the year.

[9] Our CMS and state data sources for measuring individual market exchange enrollment are different from the source we used in GAO-16-724. Our current sources measure exchange enrollment more precisely and are more complete than our prior source. That source not only included enrollment in plans sold on the exchanges, but also included enrollment in those same plans purchased off the exchanges. Therefore, the 2014 exchange enrollment data used in our prior report are not directly equivalent to the exchange enrollment data analyzed in this report.

[10] States may choose to operate their own exchanges, or this responsibility can be carried out by CMS; this responsibility can change over time. States that operate their own exchanges can use a federally facilitated exchange for certain functions, such as enrollment. We obtained data from CMS for the 39 states that used the federally facilitated exchanges for 2015, 2016, or 2017.

[11] We did not report on individual market exchange enrollment for 2014 as CMS officials had concerns with the reliability of the agency's 2014 data.

[12] From our analyses of the CMS individual market exchange enrollment data, we found that a small number of enrollees (0.3 percent of enrollees, associated with 0.2 percent of covered life-years, in the federally facilitated exchanges in 2017) appeared to have coverage from two or more issuers at the same time. Because we could not determine whether this coverage was valid, we retained the coverage in our analyses.

comparable enrollment data by rating area.[13] We used the CMS and state data to calculate the total number of issuers that participated in each state and rating area, as well as each issuer's market share—measured using covered life-years—within the state and each rating area. Rating areas represent defined localized markets within a state and issuer participation can vary across rating areas. Market concentration can vary by rating area and the largest issuer in the state may not be the largest issuer in every rating area. To account for this variability, for our analyses of the number of issuers and issuer market share in each state's individual market exchange, we calculated averages across rating areas that were weighted for differences in the size of total enrollment in each rating area. For example, to obtain the average market share of the largest issuer in a state's rating areas, we calculated the market share of the largest issuer in each rating area in the state and then calculated the average of those market shares, weighted by the number of covered life-years in each rating area.

To analyze changes in concentration in the small group exchanges— referred to as the Small Business Health Options Program (SHOP)—we obtained data from CMS and states for 2015, 2016, and 2017, the most recently available at the time of our analyses.[14] CMS provided enrollment

---

[13] We obtained data from 13 of the 14 states that operated their own individual market exchanges and did not use a federally facilitated exchange for 2015, 2016, or 2017. The remaining state, Hawaii, operated its own individual market exchange and did not use a federally facilitated exchange for 2015, but was unable to provide complete data for that year. Hawaii used a federally facilitated exchange for 2016 and 2017, so CMS provided us with data for those years. Minnesota, which operated its own individual market exchange without using a federally facilitated exchange for 2015 through 2017, was also unable to provide complete data for 2015, but provided us with data for 2016 and 2017. Officials from Hawaii and Minnesota told us that they were unable to provide 2015 data because they could not readily access historical data. Because we did not have complete individual market exchange data for 2015 through 2017 for Hawaii and Minnesota, we excluded them from our relevant findings, but provided available data for 2016 and 2017 in appendices I and II.
States generally provided enrollee member months or covered life-years for each issuer that offered plans in their individual market exchanges. Massachusetts, instead, provided the total member count for each issuer; because individuals can enroll with multiple issuers during a given year, these counts may be duplicative across issuers.

[14] We did not report on SHOP exchange enrollment data for 2014, as CMS officials stated there was no operational online data collection system in 2014. Data for 2018 were not available as the year was not complete at the time of our review. SHOP plans can begin at any time of year and generally continue for 12 months after the start date. Therefore, coverage can cross calendar years. We report SHOP exchange enrollment by calendar year, which could, therefore, include enrollment with an issuer that had exited the SHOP exchange in a given

data from its SHOP Enrollment Database for states that utilized federally facilitated SHOP exchanges operated by CMS—about two-thirds of states.[15] These data included, among other information, the coverage start and end date for each enrollee and the issuers from which the enrollees purchased coverage. Each of the remaining states operating its own exchange provided us with enrollment data for each exchange issuer.[16] We used the CMS and state data to calculate the number of issuers that participated in each state, as well as the state-level market share of each participating issuer, for each year from 2015 through 2017. SHOP exchange enrollment data at the rating area level were generally not available.

For each state's overall markets and exchanges, we counted issuers as participating in a market if they had enrollment in that market; we did not count issuers as participating if they offered coverage in a market, but did not have any enrollment. Because there can be multiple issuers within a market that share a single parent company, we aggregated such issuers to the parent company level; if there was no parent company, we analyzed the data by the individual issuers.[17] We did this to more fully account for the

---

year but is still providing coverage to enrollees whose plans began in the prior calendar year.

Our CMS and state data sources for measuring SHOP exchange enrollment are different from the source we used in GAO-16-724. Our current sources measure exchange enrollment more precisely and are more complete than our prior source.

[15] We obtained data from CMS for the 34 states that used the federally facilitated exchanges for 2015, 2016, or 2017.

[16] We obtained data from 16 of the 19 states that operated their own small group market exchanges for 2015, 2016, or 2017. Minnesota, which operated its own exchange, was unable to provide data for 2015, but provided us with data for 2016 and 2017. Utah provided issuer participation data, but was unable to provide enrollment data for 2015, 2016, or 2017. Hawaii, Idaho, and Massachusetts were unable to provide data for 2015, 2016, or 2017. Officials from Minnesota, Utah, and Massachusetts told us that they were unable to readily access historical data by issuer. Officials from Hawaii and Idaho told us that for the years in question, SHOP enrollment data was maintained by issuers, not the state. We therefore generally excluded these states from our analyses, but provided available data for these states in appendixes III and IV. States generally provided enrollee member months or covered life-years for each issuer that offered plans in their SHOP exchanges. Oregon and Washington, instead, provided us with the number of covered lives for each issuer.

[17] Specifically, we considered issuers to have the same parent company if in their Medical Loss Ratio data they reported having the same National Association of Insurance Commissioners holding group identifier, the same National Association of Insurance Commissioners

portion of the market held by each parent company. We calculated the three-firm concentration ratio—the combined shares of covered life-years for the three largest issuers in that market—and the market share of the single largest issuer in that market. We considered states' overall markets or exchanges to be highly concentrated if three or fewer issuers held at least 80 percent of the market share. Finally, while states may have multiple local markets with differing concentrations of enrollees among health issuers, the data we used to measure concentration were generally limited to enrollment at the state level, with the exception of our individual exchange enrollment data—thus precluding our ability to measure concentration within local markets except for the individual market exchanges.[18] For all other markets, we present state-wide issuer market share, although issuers may not have all participated across the entire state.

We analyzed enrollment data from all of our sources as they were reported by issuers to CMS or states. We did not otherwise independently verify the accuracy or completeness of the information with the issuers. We assessed the reliability of the CMS and state data in several ways, including through discussions with CMS and state officials, reviewing relevant data manuals and other documentation, performing electronic tests of the data to identify any outliers or anomalies, and comparing the data with data from published sources. We determined that the data were sufficiently reliable for the purposes of our reporting objectives.

We conducted this performance audit from November 2017 to March 2019 in accordance with generally accepted government auditing standards. Those standards require that we plan and perform the audit to

---

company identifier, or the same Health Insurance Oversight System company identifier. Because more recent data were not available at the time of our analysis, we relied on data from 2016 to aggregate issuers to the parent company level for 2017. CMS officials told us that the parent company relationships do not change from year to year for the majority of issuers.

[18] While the primary data sources we used in our analysis were available at the state level, we reviewed another recent analysis of concentration and found that in 39 states, the largest issuer in the state overall was also the largest issuer in at least three-quarters of the local markets studied in that state. That analysis used 2016 data on enrollment in fully and self-insured plans by metropolitan statistical areas, which include a county or counties associated with a city or urbanized area that has a population of at least 50,000. See American Medical Association, *Competition in Health Insurance: A Comprehensive Study of U.S. Markets, 2017 Update* (Chicago, IL: 2017).

obtain sufficient, appropriate evidence to provide a reasonable basis for our findings and conclusions based on our audit objectives. We believe that the evidence obtained provides a reasonable basis for our findings and conclusions based on our audit objectives.

BACKGROUND

Private health insurance is the leading source of health coverage in the United States. Small and large employers may offer fully insured group plans (by purchasing coverage from an issuer) or self-funded group plans (by setting aside funds to pay for employee health care). Most small employers purchase fully insured plans, while most large employers self-fund at least some of their employee health benefits. While the majority of health insurance coverage is provided through the small or large group market, Americans without access to group health coverage, such as those with employers that do not offer health coverage, may choose to purchase it directly from an issuer through the individual market. (See Figure 1 for total covered life-years reported by issuers to CMS in the individual and fully insured small and large group markets.)

We previously identified several factors that can affect concentration in health insurance markets.[19] High concentration levels have often been the result of consolidation—mergers and acquisitions—among existing issuers. In addition, concentration can persist because of the difficulty for new issuers to enter the market. For example, new issuers that do not yet have large numbers of enrollees may have greater challenges negotiating discounts with health care providers.

---

[19] In 2009, we conducted a structured literature review that examined the factors that can influence concentration of private health insurance markets. See GAO, *Private Health Insurance: Research on Competition in the Insurance Industry*, GAO-09-864R (Washington, D.C.: July 31, 2009).

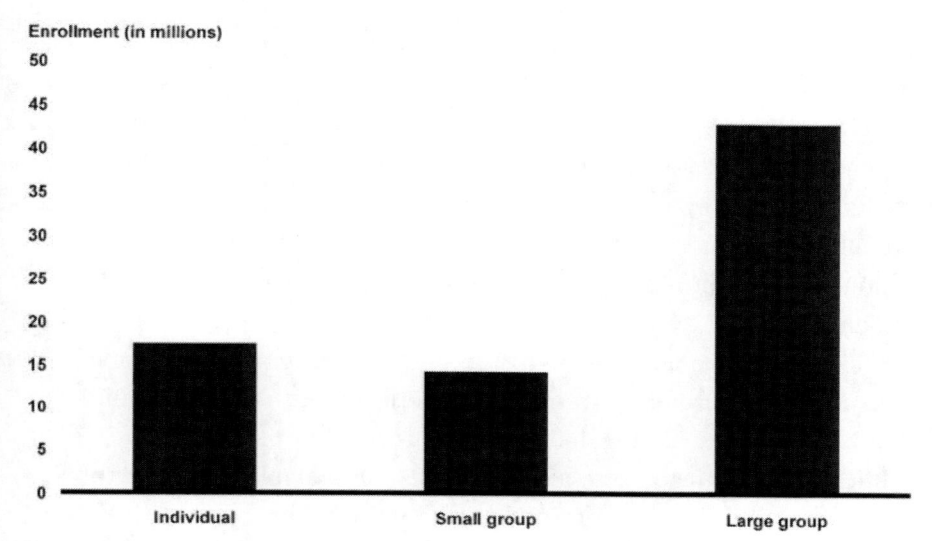

Enrollment (in millions)

Source: GAO analysis of data from the Centers for Medicare & Medicaid Services. | GAO-19-306.

Note: We calculated the size of each market using covered life-years, which measure the average number of lives insured, including dependents, during the reporting year. This is one of several ways to measure health insurance enrollment, so may differ from other measures of market size. Small and large employers may offer fully insured group plans (by purchasing coverage from an issuer) or self-funded group plans (by setting aside funds to pay for employee health care). Most small employers purchase fully insured plans, while most large employers self-fund at least some of their employee health benefits. For the small group and large group markets, enrollment data is from fully insured plans only.

Figure 1. Covered Life-Years Reported by Issuers to the Centers for Medicare & Medicaid Services in the Overall Individual, Small Group, and Large Group Health Insurance Markets, 2016.

PPACA contains provisions that may affect market concentration and competition among health issuers, such as the establishment of health insurance exchanges within each state's overall individual and small group markets. One goal of the exchanges is for issuers to have an incentive to compete with one another on price and value because consumers can visit a website to compare and select among health plans participating in the exchanges. Issuer participation in the exchanges is a key factor in assuring that consumers have a choice of health plans. While PPACA does not require issuers offering coverage in an overall market to participate in the exchanges, issuers have an incentive to do so in order to access additional consumers. For example, certain consumers earning from 100 to 400 percent of the federal poverty level are eligible to receive premium tax credits that can reduce premium costs, but only for plans purchased through an exchange.[20] The federal government and some states have also instituted other provisions to encourage issuers to participate in the exchanges.[21] For example, PPACA required the establishment of the Consumer Oriented and Operated Plan (CO-OP) program, which provided loans to new consumer-governed, nonprofit issuers that are required to offer health plans in the individual and small group exchanges.[22] In addition, in Maryland, certain issuers that offered plans outside of the exchange are also required to offer plans through the exchange. PPACA also established other key market reforms that apply both within and outside of the exchanges, such as requiring that issuers offer coverage to all individuals regardless of health status and limiting the ability of issuers to deny coverage or charge higher premiums to individuals and small groups based on health risks or certain other factors. Since the enactment of PPACA in 2010, there have been additional federal policy changes that may influence an issuer's decision about whether to participate in health insurance markets. For example, in 2014, HHS announced that a program that made payments to issuers whose losses exceeded a certain threshold— known as risk corridor payments—would be budget neutral, which resulted in reduced payments for some issuers.[23] One issuer told us that this lower

---

[20] Certain small employers may also qualify for tax credits to lower the cost of the coverage they purchase on behalf of their employees.

[21] We previously reported that most of the largest issuers in the 2012 individual and small group markets participated in the 2014 exchanges, although most of the numerous smaller issuers in those markets did not. GAO, *Patient Protection and Affordable Care Act: Largest Issuers of Health Coverage Participated in Most Exchanges, and Number of Plans Available Varied*, GAO-14-657 (Washington, D.C: Aug. 29, 2014).

[22] PPACA, § 1322, 124 Stat. at 187-192 (codified at 42 U.S.C. § 18042). By December 2012, 23 CO-OPs received federal loans to offer coverage through the individual and small group markets and all 23 CO-OPs offered plans in 2014. As of December 2018, 4 CO-OPs were still offering plans.

[23] In addition, subsequent to this announcement, legislation was enacted that prohibited CMS from paying out more in risk corridor payments than it collected for fiscal years 2015 through 2017.

than expected funding was one of multiple factors that contributed to its decision to reduce the number of insurance markets in which it participated.[24]

OVERALL INDIVIDUAL HEALTH INSURANCE MARKETS AND EXCHANGES GENERALLY REMAINED CONCENTRATED IN RECENT YEARS, WITH INCREASING CONCENTRATION IN MANY STATES' EXCHANGES

States' overall individual health insurance markets were generally concentrated in 2015 and 2016, similar to what we reported for previous years. Individual market exchanges—representing 57 percent of the overall individual market nationally in 2016—were also concentrated in most states and in many cases became more concentrated in recent years.

Overall Individual Health Insurance Markets Generally Remained Concentrated in Recent Years

States' overall individual health insurance markets were generally concentrated among a small number of issuers in 2015 and 2016. On average, there were 16 issuers participating in each state in 2016. However, that same year, the 3 largest issuers cumulatively held 80 percent or more of the market—an indicator of high concentration—in 37 of 51 states, generally consistent with what we previously reported for years 2011 through 2014 (see Figure 2).[25] The remaining issuers in each state often

---

[24] See GAO, *Health Insurance Exchanges: Claims Costs and Federal and State Policies Drove Issuer Participation, Premiums, and Plan Design*, GAO-19-215 (Washington, D.C.: Jan. 28, 2019).

[25] See GAO-16-724. See also appendix V for additional data on the overall individual market from 2011 through 2016.

In the 14 states for which the three largest issuers did not meet the 80 percent threshold, the market share of the three largest issuers varied, ranging from 42 percent in New York to 79 percent in Oregon.

had significantly smaller market shares—on average, 12 of the 16 issuers in each state held less than 5 percent market share.

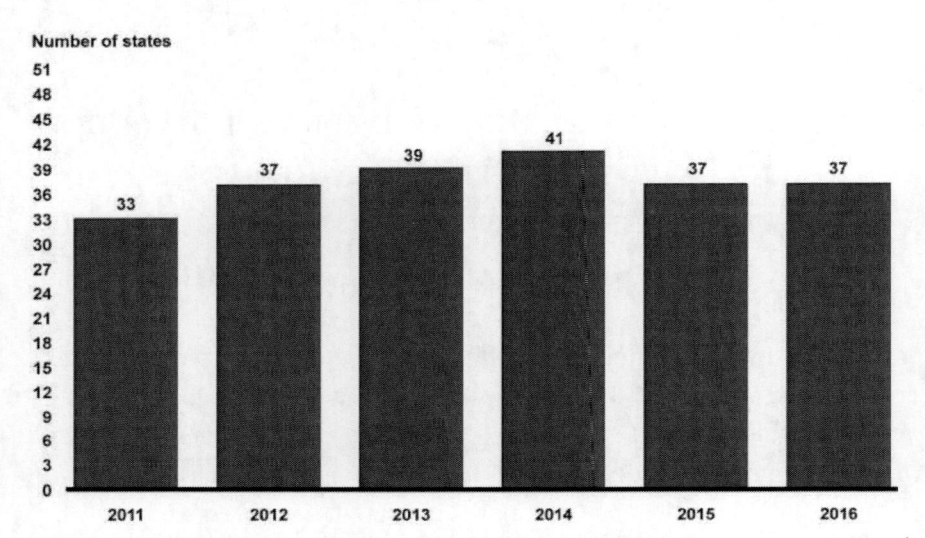

Source: GAO analysis of data from the Centers for Medicare & Medicaid Services. | GAO-19-306.

Note: This figure includes the 50 states and the District of Columbia. All states had more than three issuers in their overall individual markets during this time period. Where multiple issuers in a state shared a parent company, we aggregated the individual issuers to the parent company level. We calculated market share using covered life-years, which measure the average number of lives insured, including dependents, during the reporting year.

Figure 2. Number of States Where the Market Share of the Three Largest Issuers Was at Least 80 Percent, Overall Individual Market, 2011-2016.

We also found that in over half of states in 2016, a single issuer held at least 50 percent of the market, consistent with prior years. Specifically, a single issuer held at least 50 percent market share in 28 states in 2016. Of these states, a single issuer held between 80 and 90 percent market share in 5 states, and more than 90 percent market share in 2 states. For example, although West Virginia had 15 issuers in 2016, a single issuer, Highmark, held 91 percent market share. This largest issuer position was held by the same company in both 2015 and 2016 in 45 states; in 35 of these states, the largest issuer had been the same since 2011.

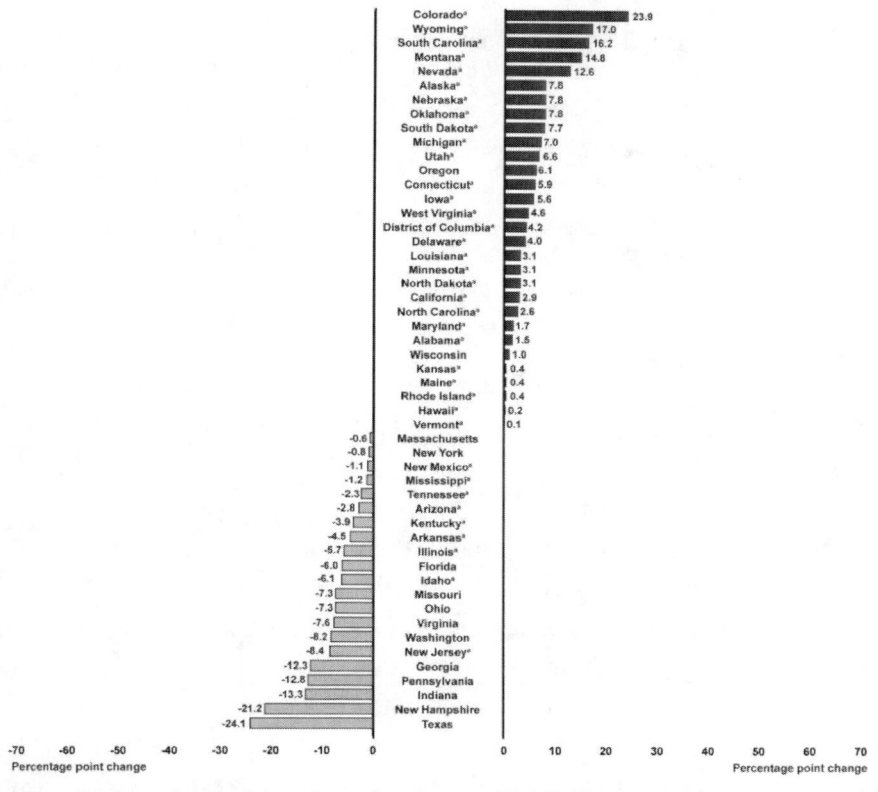

Source: GAO analysis of data from the Centers for Medicare & Medicaid Services. | GAO-19-306.

Note: This figure includes the 50 states and the District of Columbia. All states had more than three issuers in their overall individual markets during this time period. Where multiple issuers in a state shared a parent company, we aggregated the individual issuers to the parent company level. We calculated market share using covered life-years, which measure the average number of lives insured, including dependents, during the reporting year.

[a]In 2016, the three largest issuers in this state held 80 percent or more of the overall individual market.

Figure 3. Percentage Point Change in Market Share Held by the Three Largest Issuers from 2014 to 2016, by State, Overall Individual Market.

While states' overall individual markets generally remained concentrated, they experienced fluctuations in the extent of concentration in recent years. Specifically, from 2014—the last year of data on which we previously reported—to 2016, the market share of the three largest issuers increased in 30 states (with a median increase of 4 percentage points) and decreased in 21 states (with a median decrease of 6 percentage points). (See Figure 3.) However, despite these changes, states that were highly concentrated in 2014—that is, where the market share of the three largest issuers was at least 80 percent—generally remained highly concentrated in 2016.[26]

States' Individual Market Exchanges Were Generally Concentrated, and Many Became More Concentrated from 2015 to 2017

Our analyses found that states' individual market exchanges—collectively representing 57 percent of enrollment in the overall individual market nationally in 2016—were generally concentrated among a small number of issuers from 2015 to 2017.[27] Each year during this time period, for the 49 states for which we had complete data, on average, between 3 and 5 issuers participated in the individual market exchanges across the states' rating areas.[28] Further, each year, the three largest issuers held 80

---

[26] Of the 41 states that were highly concentrated in 2014, 6 states—Georgia, Indiana, New Hampshire, Pennsylvania, Texas, and Washington—were no longer highly concentrated in 2016. The market share of the three largest issuers in these states in 2016 ranged from 63 percent in Texas to 78 percent in New Hampshire. States that were not highly concentrated in 2014—that is, where the market share of the three largest issuers was less than 80 percent—were generally not highly concentrated in 2016. Of the 10 states that were not highly concentrated in 2014, 2 states—Colorado and Michigan—became highly concentrated in 2016.

[27] See appendix I for exchange enrollment as a proportion of enrollment in the overall individual market by state.

[28] Rating areas are established by states and used, in part, by issuers to set premium rates. Issuer participation and enrollment can vary across rating areas in a state. Therefore, for our analyses of issuer counts and market share within a state's individual exchange, we calculated averages across each state's rating areas and weighted the averages by the number of covered life-years in each rating area to account for variation in rating area

percent or more of the exchange market, on average, across the states' rating areas, in at least 46 states. For example, in Wisconsin in 2017, the market share of the three largest issuers ranged from 75 percent in 2 of the state's 16 rating areas to 100 percent in 6 rating areas; on average, the three largest issuers held 92 percent market share across the 16 rating areas.

While the number of states meeting this 80 percent average threshold for high concentration remained relatively constant from 2015 through 2017, market share was increasingly concentrated among a smaller number of issuers in many states, as fewer issuers participated in the exchanges by 2017.[29] The number of states with three or fewer issuers, on average, in their rating areas—and where the issuers therefore held, on average, 100 percent or nearly 100 percent market share—increased from 16 states in 2015 to 32 states in 2017.[30] (See Figure 4.)

---

enrollment. (For example, to obtain the average market share of the largest issuer in a state's rating areas, we calculated the market share of the largest issuer in each rating area in the state, then calculated the average of those market shares weighted by the number of covered life-years in each rating area.) For the purposes of this report, where we discuss average issuer counts or market share across rating areas, we are referring to these weighted averages. We did not take potential variability in issuer participation and enrollment across rating areas into account in our analyses of the overall individual, small group, or large group markets as these data were not available.

Hawaii and Minnesota are excluded from our individual market exchange analyses because we were unable to obtain data from the states for 2015. However, we present 2016 and 2017 data for these states in appendices I and II.

[29] The Kaiser Family Foundation reported in November 2018 that exchange issuer participation decreased each year between 2015 and 2018 and increased for coverage year 2019, although exchanges continued to have lower issuer participation in 2019 than in 2017 and prior years. According to the report, 608 counties nationwide gained at least one participating issuer for 2019, while 5 counties lost an issuer, as compared to 2018. (Multiple counties within a state may constitute a rating area.) Further, for coverage year 2019, fewer enrollees (17 percent of enrollees living in 37 percent of counties) have access to just one exchange issuer, as compared to the proportion of enrollees in 2018 (26 percent of enrollees living in 52 percent of counties). See Kaiser Family Foundation, *Insurer Participation on ACA Marketplaces, 2014-2019*, accessed January 17, 2019, https://www.kff.org/health-reform/issue-brief/insurer-participation-on-aca-marketplaces-20 14-2019/.

[30] The average cumulative market share of the largest one, two, or three issuers in states with three or fewer issuers, on average, was not always exactly 100 percent because states may have had more than three issuers in one or more of their rating areas. In 1 state in 2015, 2 states in 2016, and 2 states in 2017—each with three or fewer issuers, on average—the average cumulative market share of the issuers in the states was less than 100 percent, and ranged from 98 to 99 percent.

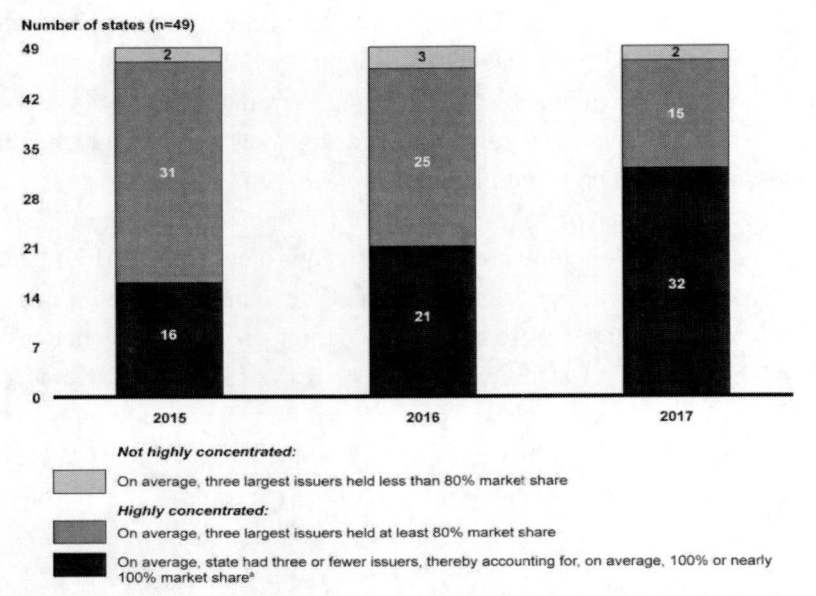

Source: GAO analysis of data from the Centers for Medicare & Medicaid Services and
states. | GAO-19-306.

Notes: We defined "highly" concentrated as three or fewer issuers holding at least 80
percent of the market share. Hawaii and Minnesota are not included in this figure
because we were unable to obtain data for all 3 years. The remaining 49 states,
including the District of Columbia, are included. Where multiple issuers in a state
shared a parent company, we aggregated the individual issuers to the parent
company level. We calculated market share using covered life-years, which
measure the average number of lives insured, including dependents, during the
reporting year. Market share in this figure refers to the average market share of the
three largest issuers across a state's rating areas, weighted by the number of
covered life-years in each rating area. Issuer counts in this figure reflect the
number of issuers, on average, across a state's rating areas, weighted by the
number of covered life-years in each rating area.

[a]The average cumulative market share of the largest one, two, or three issuers in states
with three or fewer issuers, on average, was not always exactly 100 percent
because states may have had more than three issuers in one or more of their rating
areas. In 1 state in 2015, 2 states in 2016, and 2 states in 2017—each with three or
fewer issuers, on average—the average cumulative market share of the issuers in
the states was less than 100 percent, and ranged from 98 to 99 percent.

Figure 4. Extent to Which the Three Largest Individual Market Exchange Issuers Had
at Least 80 Percent Market Share, on Average, in 49 States' Rating Areas, 2015- 2017.

Further, we found that in at least 35 states each year from 2015 through 2017, the average market share of the largest individual market exchange issuer across the states' rating areas was at least 50 percent.[31] For example, although Kansas had up to three participating exchange issuers in each of its rating areas in 2017, the largest issuer in each rating area— generally Blue Cross and Blue Shield of Kansas—had at least 88 percent market share.

We also found that many states' individual market exchanges became more concentrated from 2015 to 2017. In 32 of the 49 states, the average market share of the largest exchange issuer across the states' rating areas increased between 2015 and 2017, with a median increase of 13 percentage points. (See Figure 5.) For example:

- In Arizona, the average market share of the largest exchange issuer across the state's rating areas increased by about 60 percentage points, from 39 percent in 2015 to 98 percent in 2017. This increase corresponded with a decrease in issuer participation in the exchange; the state's seven rating areas had between 7 and 12 issuers in 2015, but by 2017 had only 1 or 2 issuers. In 2015, a CO-OP, Compass Cooperative Health Plan, Inc., had 29 percent of the total exchange market share statewide in Arizona and was among the largest issuers in three rating areas, but it exited the exchange after that year.[32] Other, smaller issuers also exited the exchange after 2015 and 2016, and, in 2017, Blue Cross Blue Shield of Arizona was left as the only issuer in five of the state's rating areas.

- In South Carolina, the average market share of the largest exchange issuer increased by 41 percentage points, from 59

---

[31] This analysis includes the states (1 in 2015, 3 in 2016, and 8 in 2017) with an average of one issuer participating in each rating area, and in which the issuers therefore had, on average, 100 percent of the market.

In 29 states, the largest issuer position at the state level was held by the same company from 2015 through 2017. However, this position was not necessarily held by the same company within each of the states' rating areas.

[32] See appendix VI for market share from 2015 through 2017 for each of the individual exchange CO-OPs.

percent in 2015 to 100 percent in 2017. As in Arizona, the increase corresponded with a decrease in issuer participation in the exchange, from 2 to 4 issuers in the state's 46 rating areas in 2015 to only 1 issuer—BlueCross BlueShield of South Carolina—in each rating area in 2017. In addition, a CO-OP, Consumers' Choice Health Insurance Company, had 43 percent of the total exchange market share statewide and was the largest issuer in nearly half of the state's rating areas in 2015, but it exited the exchange after that year. In contrast, BlueCross BlueShield of South Carolina had 42 percent of the total exchange market share statewide and was the largest issuer in about half of the rating areas in 2015, and by 2017 was the only remaining issuer in the state.

In the remaining 17 states, the average market share of the largest exchange issuer across the states' rating areas decreased between 2015 and 2017, with a median decrease of 12 percentage points. For example:

- In Maine, the average market share of the largest exchange issuer decreased by 39 percentage points, from 81 percent in 2015 to 42 percent in 2017. Maine Community Health Options, a CO-OP, remained the largest issuer in each of the state's four rating areas during this period. However, the other two issuers in these rating areas captured more market share. For instance, Harvard Pilgrim Health Care Group had 1 percent or less market share in each rating area in 2015, but as much as 32 percent market share in one of the state's rating areas in 2017.[33]

- In Delaware—which only had one rating area—the market share of the largest exchange issuer decreased by 37 percentage points, from 92 percent in 2015 to 55 percent in 2017. Although the state had the same two issuers, Aetna Group and Highmark Group, throughout this time period—and Highmark Group was the largest

---

[33] See appendix II for additional data on issuer participation and market share for the largest issuers in states' exchanges from 2015 through 2017.

issuer each year— Aetna Group's market share increased from 8 percent in 2015 to 45 percent in 2017.

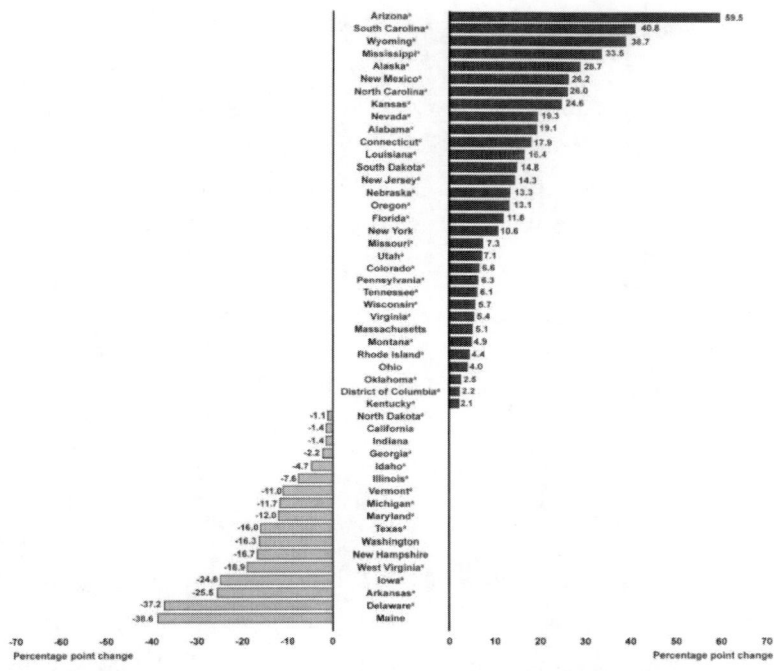

	Percentage point change
Arizona[a]	59.5
South Carolina[a]	40.8
Wyoming[a]	38.7
Mississippi[a]	33.5
Alaska[a]	28.7
New Mexico[a]	26.2
North Carolina[a]	26.0
Kansas[a]	24.6
Nevada[a]	19.3
Alabama[a]	19.1
Connecticut[a]	17.9
Louisiana[a]	16.4
South Dakota[a]	14.8
New Jersey[a]	14.3
Nebraska[a]	13.3
Oregon[a]	13.1
Florida[a]	11.8
New York	10.6
Missouri[a]	7.3
Utah[a]	7.1
Colorado[a]	6.6
Pennsylvania[a]	6.3
Tennessee[a]	6.1
Wisconsin[a]	5.7
Virginia[a]	5.4
Massachusetts	5.1
Montana[a]	4.9
Rhode Island[b]	4.4
Ohio	4.0
Oklahoma[a]	2.5
District of Columbia[a]	2.2
Kentucky[a]	2.1
North Dakota[a]	-1.1
California	-1.4
Indiana	-1.4
Georgia[a]	-2.2
Idaho[a]	-4.7
Illinois[a]	-7.6
Vermont[a]	-11.0
Michigan[a]	-11.7
Maryland[a]	-12.0
Texas[a]	-16.0
Washington	-16.3
New Hampshire	-16.7
West Virginia[a]	-18.9
Iowa[a]	-24.6
Arkansas[a]	-25.5
Delaware[a]	-37.2
Maine	-38.6

Source: GAO analysis of data from the Centers for Medicare & Medicaid Services and from states. | GAO-19-306.

Notes: Hawaii and Minnesota are not included in this figure because we were unable to obtain data for all 3 years. The remaining 49 states, including the District of Columbia, are included. Where multiple issuers in a state shared a parent company, we aggregated the individual issuers to the parent company level. We calculated issuers' market share using covered life-years, which measure the average number of lives insured, including dependents, during the reporting year. Market share refers to the average market share of the largest issuer across a state's rating areas, weighted by the number of covered life-years in each rating area. In some cases, the identity of the largest issuer varied across rating areas in a state, and changed over time.

[a]In 2017, the average market share of the largest issuer across these states' rating areas was 50 percent or more.

Figure 5. Percentage Point Change in Average Market Share of the Largest Individual Market Exchange Issuer across Rating Areas from 2015 to 2017, by State.

OVERALL SMALL GROUP HEALTH INSURANCE MARKETS AND EXCHANGES GENERALLY REMAINED CONCENTRATED IN RECENT YEARS

Our analyses found that the overall small group health insurance market remained concentrated in recent years, similar to our prior report. Small group exchanges often had low enrollment—typically less than 1 percent of the overall small group market—and also remained concentrated in recent years.

The Overall Small Group Market Remained Concentrated in Recent Years

State small group health insurance markets were concentrated among a small number of issuers in 2015 and 2016. On average, there were 8 issuers participating in each state in 2016. However, in that same year the 3 largest issuers cumulatively held 80 percent or more of the market—an indicator of high concentration—in about three-quarters of states, generally consistent with what we previously reported for years 2011 through 2014 (see Figure 6).[34] The remaining issuers in each state often had significantly smaller market shares—on average, 5 of the 8 issuers in each state held less than 5 percent market share.

Further, we found that the largest issuers held 50 percent or more of the market in 30 states in 2016. For example, though Louisiana had 6 issuers in 2016, the largest issuer held 76 percent market share. Overall, a single issuer held between 80 and 90 percent market share in 10 states, and more than 90 percent market share in 1 state. This largest issuer position was held by the same company in both 2015 and 2016 in 46 states; in 40 of these states, the largest issuer had been the same since 2011.

---

[34] See GAO-16-724. See also appendix VII for additional data on the overall small group market from 2011 through 2016.

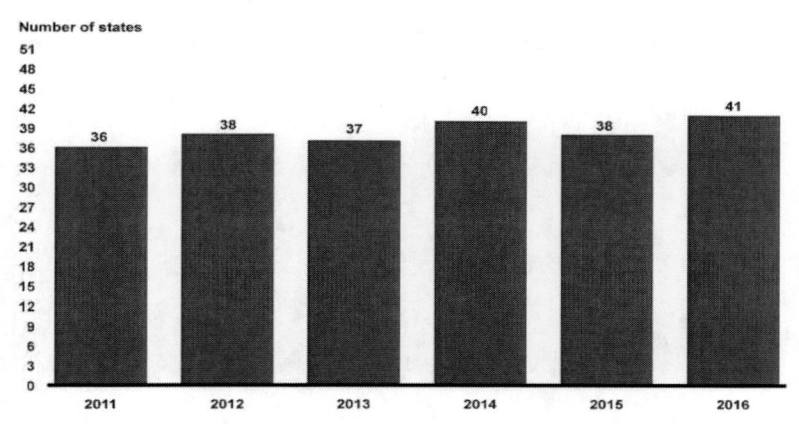

Source: GAO analysis of data from the Centers for Medicare & Medicaid Services. | GAO-19-306.

Note: This figure includes the 50 states and the District of Columbia. Three states had exactly three participating issuers in at least 1 year—Rhode Island in 2013, Delaware in 2016, and Vermont from 2012 through 2016. Therefore, these three issuers held 100 percent of the market share in those years. All other states had more than three issuers during this time period. Where multiple issuers in a state shared a parent company, we aggregated the individual issuers to the parent company level. We calculated market share using covered life-years, which measure the average number of lives insured, including dependents, during the reporting year.

Figure 6. Number of States Where the Market Share of the Three Largest Issuers Was at Least 80 Percent, Overall Small Group Market, 2011-2016.

While states' overall small group markets remained concentrated, they experienced fluctuations in concentration in recent years. From 2014 through 2016, the market share of the 3 largest issuers increased in 35 states (with a median increase of 3 percentage points), remained the same in 1 state, and decreased in 15 states (with a median decrease of 1 percentage point). (See Figure 7) However, despite these changes, states that were highly concentrated in 2014—that is, where the market share of the three largest issuers was at least 80 percent—generally remained highly concentrated in 2016.[35]

---

[35] Of the 40 states that were highly concentrated in 2014, 1 state—Connecticut—was no longer highly concentrated in 2016, where the market share of the three largest issuers was 77

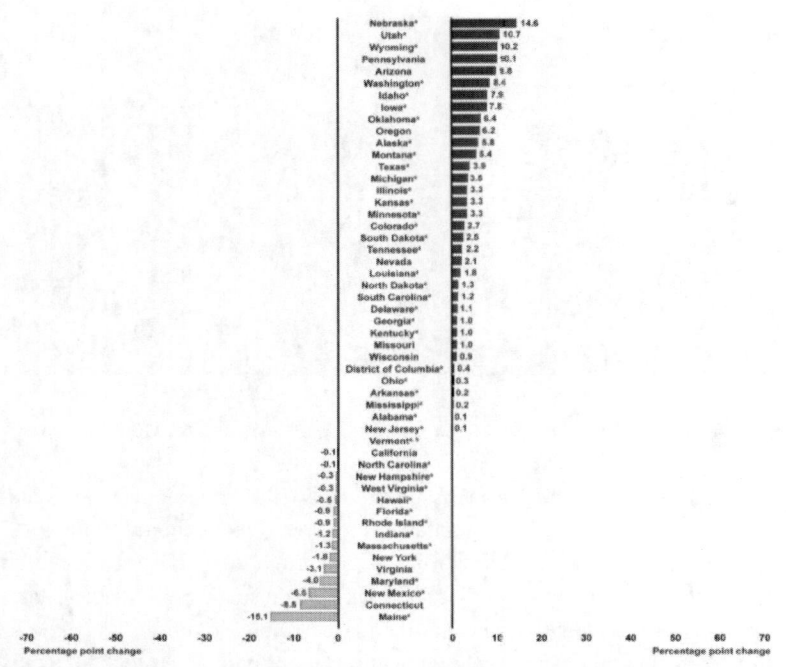

Source: GAO analysis of data from the Centers for Medicare & Medicaid Services. | GAO-19-306.

Notes: Two states had exactly three participating issuers in at least 1 year—Delaware in 2016 and Vermont from 2014 through 2016. Therefore, these three issuers held 100 percent of the market share in those years. All other states had more than three issuers from 2014 through 2016. Where multiple issuers in a state shared a parent company, we aggregated the individual issuers to the parent company level. We calculated market share using covered life-years, which measure the average number of lives insured, including dependents, during the reporting year. In some cases, the identity of the largest three issuers changed over time.

[a]In 2016, the three largest issuers in this state held 80 percent or more of the overall small group market.

[b]In Vermont there was no change in the market share held by the three largest issuers between 2014 and 2016.

Figure 7. Percentage Point Change in Market Share Held by the Three Largest Issuers from 2014 to 2016, by State, Small Group Market.

percent. States that were not highly concentrated in 2014—that is, where the market share of the three largest issuers was less than 80 percent—were generally not highly concentrated in 2016. Of the 11 states that were not highly concentrated in 2014, 2 states— Colorado and Washington—became highly concentrated in 2016.

Small Group Exchanges Were Concentrated in a Few Issuers between 2015 and 2017

Our analyses found that states' SHOP exchanges remained concentrated from 2015 to 2017, with only slight overall changes in issuer participation or market share. Further, as a proportion of the overall small group market, SHOP exchanges in most states had little enrollment. (See sidebar.)

Small Group Health Options Program (SHOP) Enrollment as a Proportion of the Overall Small Group Market

As a proportion of the overall small group market, SHOP exchanges in most states had little enrollment—that is, typically less than 1 percent of the overall small group market. For example, in 2016, Alaska's small group market had 17,257 covered life-years, while its SHOP exchange had 96 covered life-years (0.6 percent). The District of Columbia, Rhode Island, and Vermont were the only states where the SHOP exchange was more than 3 percent of the overall small group market. The District of Columbia and Vermont require all small group plans to be purchased through the state's SHOP exchange. (See app. III.)

Source: GAO. | GAO-19-306.

In each year, more than 31 of the 46 states for which we had data had three or fewer issuers in the SHOP exchange; therefore between one and three issuers held 100 percent of the market share for the state.[36] Among states with four or more issuers, the market share of the three largest issuers was typically at least 80 percent. For example, California had 6 participating issuers from 2015 through 2017 in the SHOP exchange, and the market share for the three largest issuers in that state ranged from 92 to 93 percent across the 3 years. (See Figure 8.)

---

[36] See appendix IV for additional data on issuer participation and market share for the largest issuers in states' exchanges from 2015 through 2017.

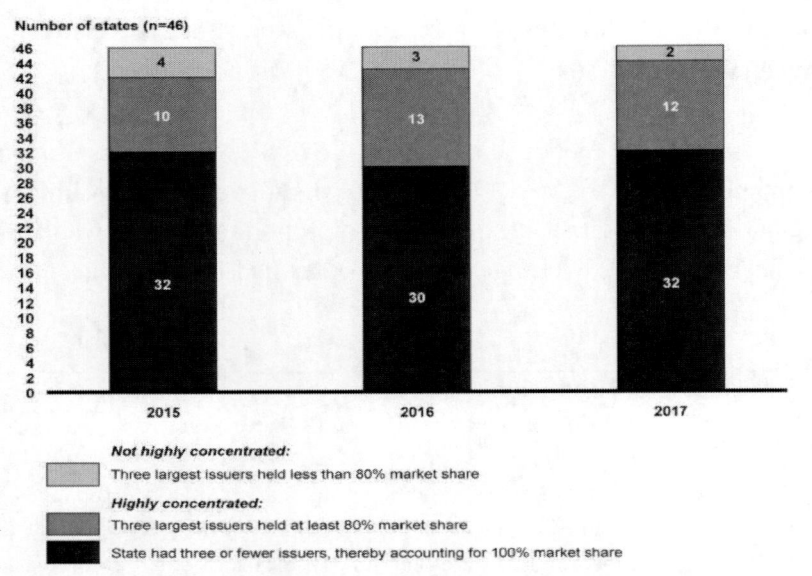

Number of states (n=46)

Source: GAO analysis of data from the Centers for Medicare & Medicaid Services and states. | GAO-19-306.

Notes: We defined "highly" concentrated as three or fewer issuers holding at least 80 percent of the market share. This figure excludes Hawaii, Idaho, Massachusetts, Minnesota, and Utah, as we did not have complete 2015 through 2017 Small Business Health Options Program data for these states. The remaining 46 states, including the District of Columbia, are included. Some states had three or fewer issuers; in these cases, all issuers—that is, one, two, or three issuers—held 100 percent of the market share. Where multiple issuers in a state shared a parent company, we aggregated the individual issuers to the parent company level. For all states other than Oregon and Washington, which provided covered lives data, we calculated market share using covered life-years, which measure the average number of lives insured, including dependents, during the reporting year.

Figure 8. Extent to Which the Three Largest Issuers Had at Least 80 Percent Market Share in 46 Small Business Health Options Program Exchanges, 2015-2017.

On average, the number of participating issuers in the SHOP exchange decreased slightly from 2015 through 2017. However, in a few states, there were larger changes in issuer participation and concentration. For example, Ohio's SHOP exchange had 7 participating issuers in 2015, decreasing to 4 issuers in 2017. Across this time period, the market share of the three largest issuers in Ohio's SHOP exchange increased from 59 percent to 98 percent. Conversely, New York's SHOP exchange had 10 issuers in 2015, decreasing to 8 issuers in 2017; but the market share of the three largest issuers decreased by almost 7 percentage points within that time.

Further, we found that in at least 38 of 46 states each year from 2015 through 2017, the largest issuer held at least 50 percent of the SHOP exchange market share. In 23 states, the market share of the largest issuer increased during this period, with a median increase of 11 percentage points, and in 6 additional states the largest issuer was the only issuer in the SHOP exchange and thus held 100 percent market share for all 3 years.[37] (See Figure 9.) For example:

- In Kentucky, the market share of the largest issuer in the SHOP exchange increased by 56 percentage points, from 42 percent in 2015 to 98 percent in 2017. In 2015, the largest issuer was Kentucky Health Cooperative, a CO-OP that exited the SHOP exchange after 2016. The second largest issuer in 2015, Wellpoint Inc. Group, increased market share over this time period, from 33 percent in 2015 to 98 percent in 2017, becoming the largest issuer. The market share of the other remaining issuer in Kentucky's SHOP exchange, Baptist Health Plan, Inc., decreased from 19 percent in 2015 to 1 percent in 2017.

- In Ohio, the market share of the largest issuer in the SHOP exchange increased by 54 percentage points, from 29 percent in 2015 to 83 percent in 2017. Across this time period, the largest issuer changed from Medical Mutual of Ohio (which had 29 percent market share in 2015 and 8 percent in 2017) to Wellpoint Inc. Group (which had 12 percent market share in 2015 and 83 percent in 2017). This increase in the largest issuer's market share corresponded with a decrease in issuer participation. The state had 7 participating issuers in 2015, decreasing to 4 in 2017. The market share of the 3 issuers that left ranged from 9 to 16 percent.

---

[37] In 33 states, the largest issuer position was held by the same company from 2015 through 2017.

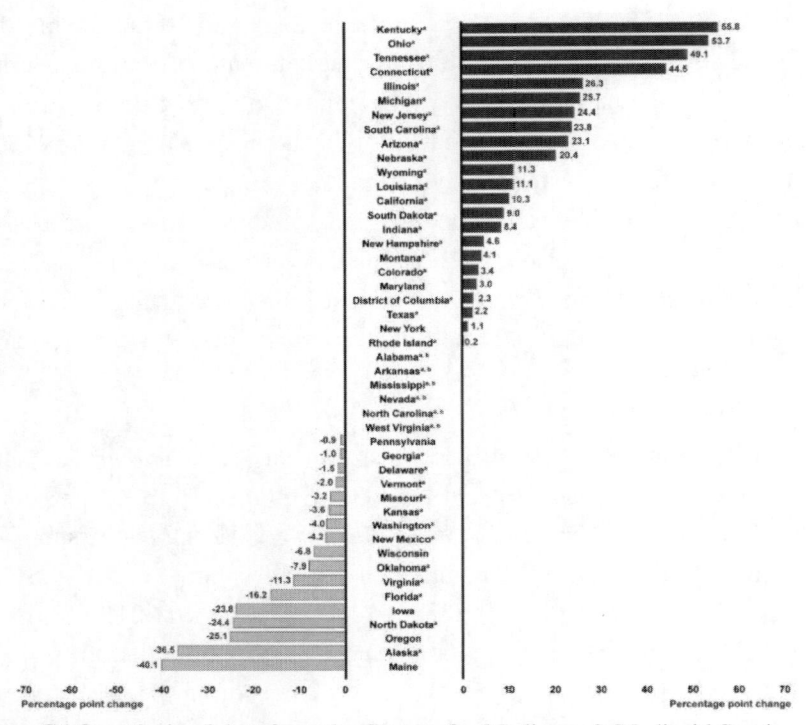

Source: GAO analysis of data from the Centers for Medicare & Medicaid Services and from states. I GAO-19-306.

Note: Hawaii, Idaho, Massachusetts, Minnesota, and Utah are not included in this figure because we were unable to obtain data for all 3 years. The remaining 46 states, including the District of Columbia, are included. Where multiple issuers in a state shared a parent company, we aggregated the individual issuers to the parent company level. For all states other than Oregon and Washington, which provided covered lives data, we calculated market share using covered life-years, which measure the average number of lives insured, including dependents, during the reporting year. In some cases, the identity of the largest issuer changed over time.

[a]In 2017, the market share of the largest issuer was 50 percent or more.

[b]In Alabama, Arkansas, Mississippi, Nevada, North Carolina, and West Virginia, the largest issuer was the only issuer in the SHOP exchange and thus held 100 percent market share between 2015 and 2017.

Figure 9. Percentage Point Change in Market Share of the Largest Small Group Exchange Issuer from 2015 to 2017 across 46 States.

In the remaining 17 states, the market share of the largest issuer decreased between 2015 and 2017, with a median decrease of 7 percentage points. In some states, these decreases were significant. For example, in Maine, the market share of the largest issuer, Maine Community Health Options—a CO-OP—decreased by 40 percentage points, from 89 percent in 2015 to 49 percent in 2017. During this time period, while Maine Community Health Options remained the largest issuer, the other two participating issuers gained additional market share. For example, Harvard Pilgrim Health Care Group increased market share from 6 percent in 2015 to 38 percent in 2017.

Overall Large Group Health Insurance Markets Remained Concentrated in Recent Years

In 2015 and 2016, states' overall large group health insurance markets remained concentrated, as in prior years.[38] On average, there were 10 participating issuers in each state in 2016. However, in that same year the 3 largest issuers held at least 80 percent market share in 43 of 51 states, which is generally consistent with prior years.[39] (See Figure 10.) In 2016, 3 issuers held 99 or 100 percent of the large group market in 7 states— Alabama, Alaska, Mississippi, Nebraska, North Dakota, South Carolina, and Vermont.[40] The remaining issuers in each state often had significantly

---

[38] The data source we analyzed for the group market only includes data on fully insured health plans. However, one survey suggests that among employers with 200 or more workers, about 80 percent of covered workers were enrolled in a self-funded plan from 2016 to 2018. (See Kaiser Family Foundation and Health Research & Educational Trust's *Employer Health Benefits Survey* for 2016, 2017, and 2018.) Therefore, the approximately 57 million covered life-years we analyzed in the large and small group markets (representing the average number of lives insured during 2016) do not represent the entire group market. Measuring enrollment another way, an estimated 178 million people had employment-based coverage at some point during 2016. (See Jessica C. Barnett and Edward R. Berchick, *Health Insurance Coverage in the United States: 2016*, Current Population Reports, P60-260, (Washington, D.C.: U.S. Government Printing Office, 2017).)

[39] Among the 8 states in which the 3 largest issuers held less than 80 percent market share, their combined market share ranged from 44 percent in Wisconsin to 79 percent in Oregon.

[40] For more on issuer participation and the market share of the largest issuers in the large group market, see app. VIII.

smaller market shares—on average, 6 of the 10 participating issuers in each state held less than 5 percent market share.

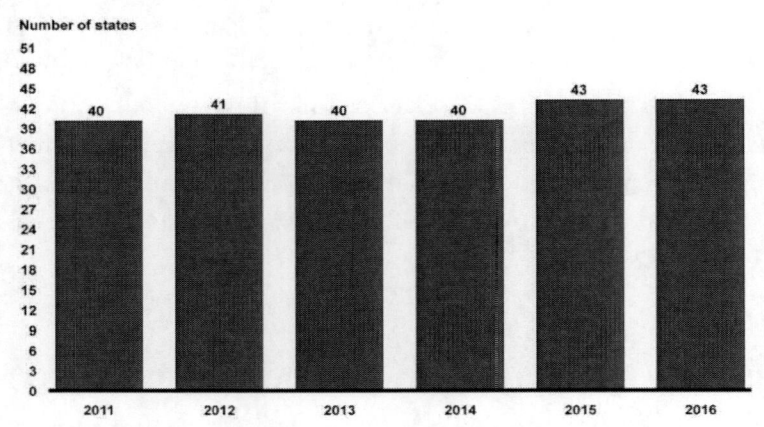

Source: GAO analysis of data from the Centers for Medicare & Medicaid Services. | GAO-19-306.

Note: This figure includes the 50 states and the District of Columbia. Vermont had exactly three participating issuers in 2012, 2015, and 2016. Therefore, the three largest issuers were the only three issuers and held 100 percent of the market share in those years. All other states had more than three issuers in each year. Where multiple issuers in a state shared a parent company, we aggregated the individual issuers to the parent company level. We calculated market share using covered life-years, which measure the average number of lives insured, including dependents, during the reporting year.

Figure 10. Number of States in Which the Three Largest Issuers Held at Least 80 Percent Market Share, Overall Large Group Market, 2011-2016.

In more than 30 states in 2015 and 2016, market share was not only concentrated among a small number of issuers, but a single issuer held at least 50 percent of the overall large group market, as in prior years. A single issuer held at least 50 percent market share in 33 states in 2016, with significantly higher levels of concentration by the largest issuer in some states. For example, in 2016, a single issuer held at least 90 percent of the market in Alabama and at least 80 percent of the market in 5 other states (Alaska, Mississippi, Montana, South Carolina, and Vermont). Further, this largest issuer position was held by the same company in 2015 and 2016 in

49 states; and, in 47 of those states, the largest issuer position has been held by the same company since 2011.

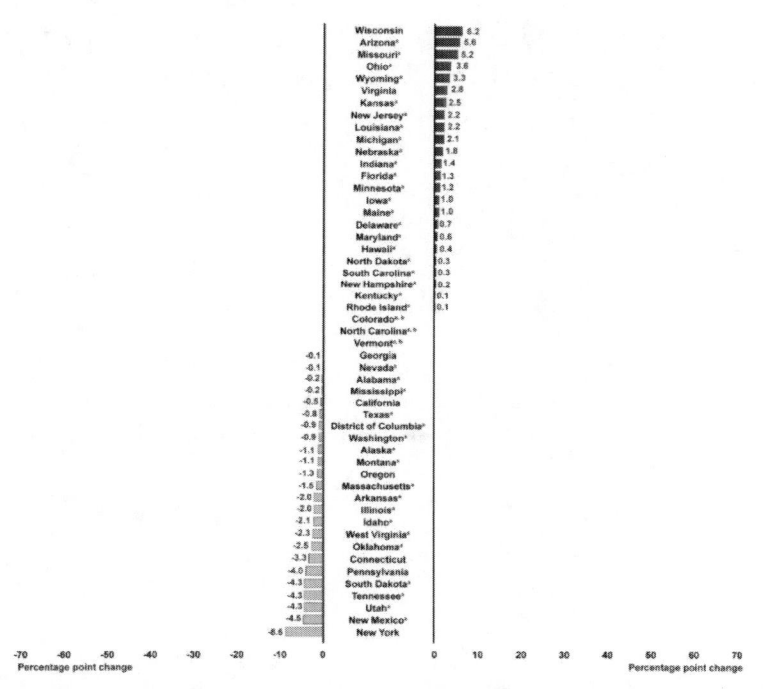

Source: GAO analysis of data from the Centers for Medicare & Medicaid Services. | GAO-19-306.

Notes: This figure includes the 50 states and the District of Columbia. Vermont had exactly three participating issuers in 2016. Therefore, the three largest issuers were the only three issuers and held 100 percent of the market share in this year. All other states had more than three issuers in each year. Where multiple issuers in a state shared a parent company, we aggregated the individual issuers to the parent company level. We calculated market share using covered life-years, which measure the average number of lives insured, including dependents, during the reporting year. In some cases, the identity of the largest three issuers changed over time.

[a]Three largest issuers in this state held at least 80 percent market share in 2016.

[b]In Colorado, North Carolina, and Vermont there was no change in the market share held by the three largest issuers between 2014 and 2016.

Figure 11. Percentage Point Change in Market Share Held by the Three Largest Issuers from 2014 to 2016, by State, Large Group Market.

The extent of concentration in the overall large group market remained relatively constant when comparing 2014—the last year of data on which we previously reported—to 2016. The market share of the 3 largest issuers increased in 24 states and decreased in 24.[41] (See Figure 11.) The largest increase was in Wisconsin, where the market share of the 3 largest issuers increased from 38 percent in 2014 to 44 percent in 2016, and the largest decrease was in New York, where the market share of the 3 largest issuers decreased from 55 percent in 2014 to 47 percent in 2016.[42]

AGENCY COMMENTS

We provided a draft of this chapter to HHS for review and comment. The department provided technical comments, which we incorporated as appropriate.

John E. Dicken
Director, Health Care

List of Committees

The Honorable Charles E. Grassley
Chairman

---

[41] Of the 40 states that were highly concentrated in 2014, 1 state was not highly concentrated in 2016: in Oregon the three largest issuers held 80 percent market share in 2014 and 79 percent market share in 2016. Of the 11 states that were not highly concentrated in 2014, 4 were highly concentrated in 2016: Arizona, Michigan, Missouri and Ohio.

[42] In accordance with federal law, in 2015, New York (along with California, Colorado, and Vermont) chose to redefine its definition of small employer from 1 to 50 employees to 1 to 100 employees, and thus employers that were previously considered part of the large group market may have instead been considered part of the small group market in 2015 and later years. See 42 U.S.C. §§ 300gg-91(e)(4), 18024(b)(2).

The Honorable Ron Wyden
Ranking Member
Committee on Finance
United States Senate

The Honorable Lamar Alexander
Chairman

The Honorable Patty Murray
Ranking Member
Committee on Health, Education, Labor, and Pensions
United States Senate

The Honorable Robert C. Scott
Chairman

The Honorable Virginia Foxx
Ranking Member
Committee on Education and Labor
House of Representatives

The Honorable Frank Pallone Jr.
Chairman

The Honorable Greg Walden
Ranking Member
Committee on Energy and Commerce
House of Representatives

The Honorable Richard Neal
Chairman

The Honorable Kevin Brady
Ranking Member
Committee on Ways and Means
House of Representatives

APPENDIX I: INDIVIDUAL MARKET HEALTH INSURANCE EXCHANGE ENROLLMENT AS A PROPORTION OF THE OVERALL MARKET, 2016

Table 1. Individual Market Health Insurance Exchange Covered Life-Years as a Proportion of Total Covered Life-Years in the Overall Individual Market, 2016

State	Covered life-years, individual market exchange	Covered life-years, overall individual market	Individual exchange covered life-years as a proportion of overall market (%)
Alabama	144,186	235,313	61.3
Alaska	15,346	21,535	71.3
Arizona	158,395	331,949	47.7
Arkansas	57,533	398,099	14.5
California	1,318,108	2,449,742	53.8
Colorado	134,133	301,117	44.6
Connecticut	85,014	176,249	48.2
Delaware	22,866	35,303	64.8
District of Columbia	17,317	20,904	82.8[a]
Florida	1,327,805	1,902,723	69.8
Georgia	410,115	594,742	69.0
Hawaii	13,323	41,383	32.2
Idaho	88,710	143,408	61.9
Illinois	300,728	620,757	48.5
Indiana	151,813	234,058	64.9
Iowa	44,554	172,995	25.8
Kansas	81,782	172,003	47.6
Kentucky	63,521	151,139	42.0
Louisiana	152,713	255,920	59.7
Maine	71,478	87,765	81.4

State	Covered life-years, individual market exchange	Covered life-years, overall individual market	Individual exchange covered life-years as a proportion of overall market (%)
Maryland	136,515	294,636	46.3
Massachusetts[b]	234,077[b]	312,591[b]	74.9[b]
Michigan	280,462	457,560	61.3
Minnesota	65,995	260,562	25.3
Mississippi	64,542	137,801	46.8
Missouri	222,775	374,187	59.5
Montana	46,803	74,953	62.4
Nebraska	73,657	149,820	49.2
Nevada	71,742	139,146	51.6
New Hampshire	45,722	104,328	43.8
New Jersey	226,492	343,272	66.0
New Mexico	42,804	71,766	59.6
New York	210,070	445,015	47.2
North Carolina	462,484	694,139	66.6
North Dakota	18,502	51,669	35.8
Ohio	191,890	385,467	49.8
Oklahoma	118,711	188,696	62.9
Oregon	121,246	231,600	52.4
Pennsylvania	370,055	600,748	61.6
Rhode Island	33,214	45,818	72.5
South Carolina	178,123	265,486	67.1
South Dakota	22,898	72,592	31.5
Tennessee	204,411	376,865	54.2
Texas	928,363	1,456,655	63.7
Utah	154,332	252,625	61.1
Vermont	26,552	31,782	83.5
Virginia	341,148	502,891	67.8
Washington	160,774	319,995	50.2
West Virginia	29,747	45,766	65.0
Wisconsin	205,923	292,340	70.4
Wyoming	20,759	31,674	65.5

Source: GAO analysis of data from the Centers for Medicare & Medicaid Services and states. | GAO-19-306.

Note: Covered life-years measure the average number of lives insured, including dependents, during the reporting year.

[a]According to exchange officials the District of Columbia requires all individual market plans to be purchased through the exchange.

[b]Massachusetts data reflect the number of covered lives, rather than covered life-years. The overall individual market count is the total number of lives insured as of the last day of the reporting year. The individual exchange count is the count of individuals enrolled in the exchange as of December 2, 2016. Counting enrollment across the year, 310,552 unique individuals were enrolled in the individual exchange in 2016.

This table presents covered life-years in each state's individual market health insurance exchange as a proportion of total covered life-years in each state's overall individual market in 2016.

APPENDIX II: NUMBER AND MARKET SHARE OF ISSUERS IN EACH STATE'S INDIVIDUAL MARKET HEALTH INSURANCE EXCHANGE, 2015-2017

The four tables below present information on the number of participating issuers and market share of the largest issuers in each state's individual market exchange from 2015 through 2017. Specifically, Table 2 presents the total number of exchange issuers in each state. Table 3 presents the average number of exchange issuers across each state's rating areas. Table 4 presents the names and market shares of the single largest exchange issuer, and market share of the largest three issuers, for each state. Table 5 presents the average market share of the largest issuer across each state's rating areas.

Table 2. Number of Issuers in Each State's Individual Market Health Insurance Exchange, 2015-2017

State	Number of issuers (2015)	Number of issuers (2016)	Number of issuers (2017)
Alabama	3	3	1
Alaska	2	2	1
Arizona	12	8	2
Arkansas	4	5	4
California	10	12	11
Colorado	10	8	7
Connecticut	4	4	2
Delaware	2	2	2
District of Columbia	3	2	2
Florida	11	7	5
Georgia	9	8	5
Hawaii	a	2	2
Idaho	5	5	5

State	Number of issuers (2015)	Number of issuers (2016)	Number of issuers (2017)
Illinois	8	7	5
Indiana	9	8	4
Iowa	4	4	4
Kansas	3	3	3
Kentucky	5	7	3
Louisiana	5	4	3
Maine	3	3	3
Maryland	5	5	3
Massachusetts	10	10	9
Michigan	13	11	9
Minnesota	a	4	4
Mississippi	3	3	2
Missouri	6	6	4
Montana	4	3	3
Nebraska	4	4	2
Nevada	5	3	3
New Hampshire	5	5	4
New Jersey	5	5	2
New Mexico	5	4	4
New York	16	15	14
North Carolina	3	3	2
North Dakota	3	3	3
Ohio	16	15	10
Oklahoma	4	2	1
Oregon	10	10	6
Pennsylvania	9	8	5
Rhode Island	3	3	2
South Carolina	4	3	1
South Dakota	3	2	2
Tennessee	5	4	3
Texas	14	16	10
Utah	6	4	3
Vermont	2	2	2
Virginia	7	9	10
Washington	9	10	8
West Virginia	1	2	2
Wisconsin	15	15	14
Wyoming	2	1	1

Source: GAO analysis of data from the Centers for Medicare & Medicaid Services and states. | GAO-19-306.

Note: Where multiple issuers in a state shared a parent company, we aggregated the individual issuers to the parent company level.

aData were not available from Hawaii or Minnesota for 2015.

Table 3. Average Number of Individual Market Health Insurance Exchange Issuers Participating in a State's Rating Areas, by State, 2015-2017

State	Weighted average number of issuers participating in states' rating areas (2015)	Weighted average number of issuers participating in states' rating areas (2016)	Weighted average number of issuers participating in states' rating areas (2017)
Alabama	2.3	2.4	1.0
Alaska	2.0	2.0	1.0
Arizona	11.0	6.3	1.2
Arkansas	3.7	5.0	3.9
California	4.8	5.3	5.3
Colorado	8.2	6.7	4.9
Connecticut	4.0	4.0	2.0
Delaware	2.0	2.0	2.0
District of Columbia	3.0	2.0	2.0
Florida	6.1	4.4	2.9
Georgia	7.8	6.9	3.9
Hawaii	a	2.0	2.0
Idaho	5.0	5.0	5.0
Illinois	5.7	5.2	2.6
Indiana	6.9	6.7	3.9
Iowa	2.6	3.4	3.4
Kansas	2.4	2.4	2.4
Kentucky	4.8	6.4	2.3
Louisiana	4.1	3.5	2.5
Maine	3.0	3.0	3.0
Maryland	5.0	5.0	3.0
Massachusetts	9.9	10.0	9.0
Michigan	7.6	6.2	6.2
Minnesota	a	3.7	3.3
Mississippi	2.9	2.9	1.9
Missouri	3.3	3.7	2.0
Montana	4.0	3.0	3.0
Nebraska	3.9	4.0	2.0
Nevada	4.1	2.9	2.9

State	Weighted average number of issuers participating in states' rating areas (2015)	Weighted average number of issuers participating in states' rating areas (2016)	Weighted average number of issuers participating in states' rating areas (2017)
New Hampshire	5.0	5.0	4.0
New Jersey	5.0	5.0	2.0
New Mexico	5.0	4.0	4.0
New York	10.0	8.8	8.9
North Carolina	2.7	2.7	1.3
North Dakota	3.0	3.0	3.0
Ohio	10.0	9.8	4.9
Oklahoma	3.6	2.0	1.0
Oregon	8.2	7.7	4.6
Pennsylvania	4.9	4.0	2.0
Rhode Island	3.0	3.0	2.0
South Carolina	3.6	1.7	1.0
South Dakota	3.0	2.0	2.0
Tennessee	4.1	3.1	1.5
Texas	7.7	7.3	3.5
Utah	5.3	3.1	2.8
Vermont	2.0	2.0	2.0
Virginia	4.4	5.6	5.4
Washington	7.3	7.7	6.6
West Virginia	1.0	1.3	1.8
Wisconsin	6.3	6.9	5.1
Wyoming	2.0	1.0	1.0

Source: GAO analysis of data from the Centers for Medicare & Medicaid Services and states. | GAO-19-306.

Note: Where multiple issuers in a state shared a parent company, we aggregated the individual issuers to the parent company level. Rating areas are established by states and used, in part, by issuers to set premium rates. Issuer participation and enrollment can vary across rating areas in a state. The issuer counts in this table reflect the average number of participating issuers across a state's rating areas, weighted by the number of covered life-years in each rating area.

[a]Data were not available from Hawaii or Minnesota for 2015.

Table 4. Market Share of the Single Largest and Three Largest Issuers in Each State's Individual Market Health Insurance Exchange, 2015-2017

State	Name	Market share of single largest issuer (%) 2015	Market share of single largest issuer (%) 2016	Market share of single largest issuer (%) 2017	Market share of the largest three issuers (%) 2015	Market share of the largest three issuers (%) 2016	Market share of the largest three issuers (%) 2017
Alabama	BCBS OF AL GRP	80.9	67.3	100.0	100.0	100.0	100.0
Alaska	OREGON DENTAL GRP	71.3	69.8	not the largest	100.0	100.0	100.0
Alaska	PREMERA BLUE CROSS GROUP	not the largest	not the largest	100.0	100.0	100.0	100.0
Arizona	CENTENE CORP GRP	32.4	not the largest	72.6	80.8	76.3	100.0
Arizona	UNITEDHEALTH GRP	not the largest	37.6	not the largest	80.8	76.3	100.0
Arkansas	ARKANSAS BCBS GRP	94.2	91.9	68.7	100.0	99.2	99.9
California	WELLPOINT INC GRP	27.8	not the largest	not the largest	78.2	78.5	72.4
California	BLUE SHIELD OF CALIFORNIA GROUP	not the largest	30.0	not the largest	78.2	78.5	72.4
California	KAISER FOUNDATION GRP	not the largest	not the largest	28.3	78.2	78.5	72.4
Colorado	COLORADO HEALTH INSURANCE COOPERATIVE, INC.	43.0	not the largest	not the largest	85.6	78.5	89.9

State	Name	Market share of single largest issuer (%) 2015	Market share of single largest issuer (%) 2016	Market share of single largest issuer (%) 2017	Market share of the largest three issuers (%) 2015	Market share of the largest three issuers (%) 2016	Market share of the largest three issuers (%) 2017
Connecticut	HIP INS GRP	43.1	50.6	63.4	97.8	97.8	100.0
Delaware	HIGHMARK GRP	91.9	90.5	54.7	100.0	100.0	100.0
District of Columbia	CAREFIRST INC GRP	80.8	85.6	83.0	100.0	100.0	100.0
Florida	BLUE CROSS AND BLUE SHIELD OF FLORIDA, INC.	26.3	40.1	58.9	66.1	72.5	97.4
Georgia	HUMANA GRP	56.7	32.4	not the largest	84.9	68.9	93.1
Georgia	WELLPOINT INC GRP	not the largest	not the largest	48.1	84.9	68.9	93.1
Hawaii	HAWAII MEDICAL SERVICE ASSOCIATION	a	58.6	52.8	a	100.0	100.0
Idaho	BLUE CROSS OF IDAHO HEALTH SERVICE, INC.	56.7	43.7	not the largest	98.7	91.8	85.8
Idaho	IHC INC GRP	not the largest	not the largest	36.1	98.7	91.8	85.8
Illinois	HCSC GRP	77.4	57.1	66.0	94.4	77.3	90.7
Indiana	WELLPOINT INC GRP	47.0	30.4	not the largest	74.7	66.1	80.3
Indiana	CENTENE CORP GRP	not the largest	not the largest	35.6	74.7	66.1	80.3
Iowa	AETNA GRP	97.4	72.8	67.0	99.9	99.8	99.2
Kansas	AETNA GRP	55.6	not the largest	not the largest	100.0	100.0	100.0

Table 4. (Continued)

State	Name	Market share of single largest issuer (%) 2015	Market share of single largest issuer (%) 2016	Market share of single largest issuer (%) 2017	Market share of the three largest issuers (%) 2015	Market share of the three largest issuers (%) 2016	Market share of the three largest issuers (%) 2017
Kansas	BCBS OF KS GRP	not the largest	62.2	61.3	100.0	100.0	100.0
Kentucky	KENTUCKY HEALTH COOPERATIVE	64.3	not the largest	not the largest	93.7	87.5	100.0
Kentucky	WELLPOINT INC GRP	not the largest	62.7	59.8	93.7	87.5	100.0
Louisiana	LOUISIANA HLTH SERV GRP	53.3	47.9	68.2	89.1	89.3	100.0
Maine	MAINE COMMUNITY HEALTH OPTIONS	81.0	67.5	42.4	100.0	100.0	100.0
Maryland	CAREFIRST INC GRP	77.5	64.6	65.4	96.9	93.2	100.0
Massachusetts	TUFTS HEALTH PLAN	40.6	46.8	47.1	82.5	86.9	90.5
Michigan	BCBS OF MI GRP	67.5	55.5	49.5	88.0	87.8	86.0
Minnesota	BCBS OF MN GRP	a	27.9	not the largest	a	78.5	76.8
Minnesota	HEALTHPARTNERS GRP	a	not the largest	26.0	a	78.5	76.8
Mississippi	HUMANA GRP	38.2	not the largest	not the largest	100.0	100.0	100.0
Mississippi	CENTENE CORP GRP	not the largest	50.3	90.4	100.0	100.0	100.0

State	Name	Market share of single largest issuer (%) 2015	Market share of single largest issuer (%) 2016	Market share of single largest issuer (%) 2017	Market share of the largest three issuers (%) 2015	Market share of the largest three issuers (%) 2016	Market share of the largest three issuers (%) 2017
Missouri	AETNA GRP	58.3	35.6	not the largest	86.2	71.2	91.9
Missouri	WELLPOINT INC GRP	not the largest	not the largest	44.7	86.2	71.2	91.9
Montana	HCSC GRP	46.1	61.5	43.5	98.2	100.0	100.0
Nebraska	AETNA GRP	60.4	47.8	56.0	96.5	93.9	100.0
Nevada	UNITEDHEALTH GRP	42.5	56.1	56.6	86.9	100.0	100.0
New Hampshire	WELLPOINT INC GRP	60.2	46.0	not the largest	92.7	96.0	99.8
New Hampshire	MINUTEMAN HEALTH, INC	not the largest	not the largest	43.5	92.7	96.0	99.8
New Jersey	BCBS OF NJ GRP	54.0	60.1	68.3	95.5	89.9	100.0
New Mexico	HCSC GRP	40.3	not the largest	not the largest	89.1	93.4	97.0
New Mexico	MOLINA HEALTHCARE INC GRP	not the largest	40.0	62.0	89.1	93.4	97.0
New York	NEW YORK STATE CATHOLIC HEALTH PLAN, INC.	19.5	26.2	32.9	47.3	47.0	55.3
North Carolina	BLUE CROSS AND BLUE SHIELD OF NORTH CAROLINA	67.3	46.5	95.6	100.0	100.0	100.0

Table 4. (Continued)

State	Name	Market share of single largest issuer (%) 2015	Market share of single largest issuer (%) 2016	Market share of single largest issuer (%) 2017	Market share of the largest three issuers (%) 2015	Market share of the largest three issuers (%) 2016	Market share of the largest three issuers (%) 2017
North Dakota	NORIDIAN MUTUAL INSURANCE COMPANY	69.0	54.0	71.1	100.0	100.0	100.0
Ohio	MEDICAL MUTUAL OF OHIO	27.0	not the largest	not the largest	61.3	63.2	74.3
Ohio	CARESOURCE MANAGEMENT GROUP	not the largest	28.8	31.7	61.3	63.2	74.3
Oklahoma	HCSC GRP	97.5	94.9	100.0	99.8	100.0	100.0
Oregon	OREGON DENTAL GRP	41.9	not the largest	not the largest	80.3	82.5	82.0
Oregon	PROVIDENCE HEALTH PLAN	not the largest	51.2	50.4	80.3	82.5	82.0
Pennsylvania	HIGHMARK GRP	46.1	not the largest	not the largest	81.4	67.1	77.3
Pennsylvania	INDEPENDENCE HEALTH GROUP, INC.		31.0	39.4	81.4	67.1	77.3
Rhode Island	NEIGHBORHOOD HEALTH PLAN OF RHODE ISLAND	50.1	not the largest	54.5	100.0	100.0	100.0
Rhode Island	BLUE CROSS & BLUE SHIELD OF RHODE ISLAND	not the largest	48.5	not the largest	100.0	100.0	100.0

State	Name	Market share of single largest issuer (%) 2015	Market share of single largest issuer (%) 2016	Market share of single largest issuer (%) 2017	Market share of the largest three issuers (%) 2015	Market share of the largest three issuers (%) 2016	Market share of the largest three issuers (%) 2017
South Carolina	CONSUMERS' CHOICE HEALTH INSURANCE COMPANY	42.5	not the largest	not the largest	99.7	100.0	100.0
South Carolina	BCBS OF SC GRP	not the largest	95.5	100.0	99.7	100.0	100.0
South Dakota	AVERA HEALTH PLANS, INC.	52.9	73.2	75.5	100.0	100.0	100.0
Tennessee	BCBS OF TN INC	77.6	65.6	35.2	99.3	92.3	100.0
Texas	HCSC GRP	64.9	39.6	27.8	84.7	63.5	73.6
Utah	IHC INC GRP	49.1	61.9	55.2	82.7	99.1	100.0
Vermont	BCBS OF VT GRP	91.7	88.0	80.7	100.0	100.0	100.0
Virginia	WELLPOINT INC GRP	39.8	38.2	43.6	71.9	67.8	74.3
Washington	PREMERA BLUE CROSS GROUP	48.5	39.1	not the largest	82.7	75.0	68.2
Washington	MOLINA HEALTHCARE INC GRP	not the largest	not the largest	23.4	82.7	75.0	68.2
West Virginia	HIGHMARK GRP	100.0	95.9	79.4	100.0	100.0	100.0
Wisconsin	COMMON GROUND HEALTHCARE COOPERATIVE	17.1	not the largest	not the largest	46.7	57.6	58.7

Table 4. (Continued)

State	Name	Market share of single largest issuer (%) 2015	Market share of single largest issuer (%) 2016	Market share of single largest issuer (%) 2017	Market share of the largest three issuers (%) 2015	Market share of the largest three issuers (%) 2016	Market share of the largest three issuers (%) 2017
Wisconsin	MOLINA HEALTHCARE INC GRP	not the largest	28.4	31.0	46.7	57.6	58.7
Wyoming	BLUE CROSS BLUE SHIELD OF WYOMING	58.3	100.0	100.0	100.0	100.0	100.0

Legend: — This symbol indicates that this issuer was not the largest in that year.

Source: GAO analysis of data from the Centers for Medicare & Medicaid Services and states. │GAO-19-306.

Note: Where multiple issuers in a state shared a parent company, we aggregated the individual issuers to the parent company level. We measured issuers' market share using covered life-years, which measure the average number of lives insured, including dependents, during the reporting year. Market share in this table represents an issuer's total state-level market share, which does not take into account variations in market share across a state's exchange rating areas. We reprinted issuer names as they were reported in the data from the Centers for Medicare & Medicaid Services.

[a]Data were not available from Hawaii or Minnesota for 2015.

Table 5. Average Market Share of the Largest Issuer across a State's Rating Areas, Individual Market Health Insurance Exchanges, 2015-2017

State	Weighted average market share of the largest issuer across states' rating areas (2015)	Weighted average market share of the largest issuer across states' rating areas (2016)	Weighted average market share of the largest issuer across states' rating areas (2017)
Alabama	80.9	68.0	100.0
Alaska	71.3	69.8	100.0
Arizona	38.8	42.3	98.3
Arkansas	94.2	91.9	68.7
California	43.4	42.9	42.0
Colorado	48.5	54.3	55.1
Connecticut	54.8	62.8	72.7
Delaware	91.9	90.5	54.7
District of Columbia	80.8	85.6	83.0
Florida	58.7	62.0	70.5
Georgia	60.7	38.1	58.5
Hawaii	a	58.6	52.8
Idaho	60.5	48.8	55.8
Illinois	78.4	61.1	70.9
Indiana	47.8	32.5	46.4
Iowa	97.4	75.5	72.6
Kansas	66.1	82.7	90.7
Kentucky	65.3	63.4	67.4
Louisiana	53.3	49.9	69.7
Maine	81.0	67.5	42.4
Maryland	77.5	64.6	65.4
Massachusetts	42.0	47.1	47.1
Michigan	67.7	57.9	56.0
Minnesota	a	44.1	51.0
Mississippi	56.9	54.3	90.4
Missouri	66.3	51.9	73.6
Montana	46.8	61.5	51.7
Nebraska	60.4	47.8	73.7
Nevada	47.9	63.4	67.2
New Hampshire	60.2	46.0	43.5
New Jersey	54.0	60.1	68.3

Table 5. (Continued)

State	Weighted average market share of the largest issuer across states' rating areas (2015)	Weighted average market share of the largest issuer across states' rating areas (2016)	Weighted average market share of the largest issuer across states' rating areas (2017)
New Mexico	42.6	43.6	68.8
New York	24.8	28.4	35.4
North Carolina	69.6	60.4	95.6
North Dakota	72.2	60.3	71.1
Ohio	41.1	39.2	45.1
Oklahoma	97.5	94.9	100.0
Oregon	41.9	55.6	55.0
Pennsylvania	73.3	64.4	79.6
Rhode Island	50.1	48.5	54.5
South Carolina	59.2	95.5	100.0
South Dakota	60.7	73.2	75.5
Tennessee	77.6	65.6	83.7
Texas	69.4	43.5	53.3
Utah	54.5	61.9	61.6
Vermont	91.7	88.0	80.7
Virginia	51.2	50.7	56.6
Washington	48.5	40.4	32.2
West Virginia	100.0	95.9	81.1
Wisconsin	51.8	54.1	57.5
Wyoming	61.3	100.0	100.0

Source: GAO analysis of data from the Centers for Medicare & Medicaid Services and states. | GAO-19-306.

Note: Where multiple issuers in a state shared a parent company, we aggregated the individual issuers to the parent company level. We calculated issuers' market share using covered life-years, which measure the average number of lives insured, including dependents, during the reporting year. Rating areas are established by states and used, in part, by issuers to set premium rates. Issuer participation and enrollment can vary across rating areas in a state. The market shares in this table reflect the average market share of the largest issuer across a state's rating areas, weighted by the number of covered life-years in each rating area. In some cases, the identity of the largest issuer varied across rating areas in a state and changed over time.

[a]Data were not available from Hawaii or Minnesota for 2015.

APPENDIX III: SMALL GROUP HEALTH INSURANCE EXCHANGE ENROLLMENT AS A PROPORTION OF THE OVERALL MARKET, 2016

This table presents covered life-years in each state's Small Business Health Options Program (SHOP) exchange as a proportion of total covered life-years in each state's overall small group market in 2016.

Table 6. Small Business Health Options Program (SHOP) Exchange Covered Life-Years as a Proportion of Total Covered Life-Years in the Overall Small Group Market, 2016

State	Covered life-years, SHOP exchange	Covered life-years overall small group market	SHOP exchange covered life-years as a proportion of overall market (%)
Alabama	673	218,406	0.3
Alaska	96	17,257	0.6
Arizona	968	172,243	0.6
Arkansas	340	100,328	0.3
California	18,863	2,269,783	0.8
Colorado	2,977	240,514	1.2
Connecticut	1,476	166,597	0.9
Delaware	202	31,158	0.7
District of Columbia	26,356	89,280	29.5[a]
Florida	1,827	610,617	0.3
Georgia	948	253,257	0.4
Illinois	2,502	525,560	0.5
Indiana	264	189,262	0.1
Iowa	70	158,272	0.0
Kansas	1,573	140,187	1.1
Kentucky	258	125,044	0.2
Louisiana	441	193,777	0.2
Maine	718	64,342	1.1
Maryland[b]	397	256,684	0.2
Michigan	1,790	449,905	0.4
Minnesota	1,894	265,555	0.7
Mississippi	213	88,294	0.2
Missouri	791	238,515	0.3
Montana	1,061	46,939	2.3

Table 6. (Continued)

State	Covered life-years, SHOP exchange	Covered life-years overall small group market	SHOP exchange covered life-years as a proportion of overall market (%)
Nebraska	176	76,140	0.2
Nevada	76	90,111	0.1
New Hampshire	778	70,891	1.1
New Jersey	1,166	449,474	0.3
New Mexico	1,307	51,881	2.5
New York	13,015	1,180,566	1.1
North Carolina	1,356	271,353	0.5
North Dakota	143	59,757	0.2
Ohio	758	676,460	0.1
Oklahoma	1,002	178,940	0.6
Oregon[c]	1,557[c]	185,676[c]	0.8[c]
Pennsylvania	3,592	651,671	0.6
Rhode Island	4,313	57,111	7.6
South Carolina	510	111,083	0.5
South Dakota	125	52,609	0.2
Tennessee	552	286,983	0.2
Texas	4,250	956,157	0.4
Vermont	46,396	46,789	99.2[a]
Virginia	1,645	355,498	0.5
Washington[c]	1,557[c]	288,355[c]	0.5[c]
West Virginia	436	42,234	1.0
Wisconsin	1,270	277,642	0.5
Wyoming	166	18,675	0.9

Source: GAO analysis of data from the Centers for Medicare & Medicaid Services and states. | GAO-19-306.

Notes: This table excludes Hawaii, Idaho, Massachusetts, and Utah, as we did not have 2016 SHOP enrollment data for these states. We calculated market share using covered life-years, which measure the average number of lives insured, including dependents, during the reporting year.

[a]The District of Columbia and Vermont require all small group plans to be purchased through the state's SHOP exchange. According to officials, in July 2016, the District of Columbia began converting all small group plans onto the state's SHOP exchange, and continued this conversion process monthly through June 2017 as plans came up for renewal.

[b]According to Maryland officials, although partial data from all issuers is included, the 2016 exchange enrollment total may be an undercount because of a transition in the data collection process.

[c]Data from Oregon and Washington reflect the number of covered lives, rather than covered life-years. The overall small group market count is the total number of lives insured as of the last day of the reporting year.

APPENDIX IV: NUMBER AND MARKET SHARE OF ISSUERS IN EACH STATE'S SMALL GROUP HEALTH INSURANCE EXCHANGE, 2015-2017

The two tables below present information on the participation of issuers in each state's small group health insurance exchange from 2015 to 2017 and the market share of the largest and three largest issuers from 2015 to 2017.

Table 7. Number of Issuers in Each State's Small Group Health Insurance Exchange, 2015-2017

State	Number of issuers (2015)	Number of issuers (2016)	Number of issuers (2017)
Alabama	1	1	1
Alaska	2	2	2
Arizona	5	4	3
Arkansas	1	1	1
California	6	6	6
Colorado	6	4	4
Connecticut	3	3	3
Delaware	2	2	2
District of Columbia	4	4	4
Florida	4	5	5
Georgia	3	4	4
Illinois	3	3	2
Indiana	2	2	1
Iowa	3	3	3
Kansas	2	2	2
Kentucky	4	4	3
Louisiana	3	2	2
Maine	3	3	3
Maryland	5	5	5
Michigan	6	5	4
Minnesota	[a]	1	1

Table 7. (Continued)

State	Number of issuers (2015)	Number of issuers (2016)	Number of issuers (2017)
Mississippi	1	1	1
Missouri	2	2	2
Montana	3	3	3
Nebraska	2	1	1
Nevada	1	1	1
New Hampshire	4	4	4
New Jersey	2	3	2
New Mexico	3	3	3
New York	10	8	8
North Carolina	1	1	1
North Dakota	3	3	2
Ohio	7	7	4
Oklahoma	3	3	2
Oregon	8	7	5
Pennsylvania	6	7	7
Rhode Island	3	3	3
South Carolina	2	1	1
South Dakota	3	2	2
Tennessee	2	1	1
Texas	3	3	3
Utah	3	3	2
Vermont	2	2	2
Virginia	3	4	4
Washington	3	3	2
West Virginia	1	1	1
Wisconsin	9	9	8
Wyoming	2	1	1

Source: GAO analysis of data from the Centers for Medicare & Medicaid Services and states. | GAO-19-306.

Note: This table excludes Hawaii, Idaho, and Massachusetts, as we did not have SHOP data for these states. Where multiple issuers in a state shared a parent company, we aggregated the individual issuers to the parent company level.

[a]Data were not available from Minnesota for 2015.

Table 8. Market Share of the Single Largest and Three Largest Issuers in Each State's Small Group Health Insurance Exchange, 2015-2017

State	Name	Market share of the largest single issuer (%) (2015)	Market share of the largest single issuer (%) (2016)	Market share of the largest single issuer (%) (2017)	Market share of the largest three issuers (%) (2015)	Market share of the largest three issuers (%) (2016)	Market share of the largest three issuers (%) (2017)
Alabama	BCBS OF AL GRP	100.0	100.0	100.0	100.0	100.0	100.0
Alaska	OREGON DENTAL GRP	86.7	78.6	50.2	100.0	100.0	100.0
Arizona	CENTENE CORP GRP	64.8	62.3	not the largest	93.3	100.0	100.0
Arizona	BLUE CROSS AND BLUE SHIELD OF ARIZONA, INC.	not the largest	not the largest	88.0			
Arkansas	ARKANSAS BCBS GRP	100.0	100.0	100.0	100.0	100.0	100.0
California	KAISER FOUNDATION GRP	58.7	66.0	69.0	93.2	92.2	92.2
Colorado	KAISER FOUNDATION GRP	54.0	62.6	57.4	85.9	98.9	97.7
Connecticut	WELLPOINT INC GRP	52.5	48.0	97.0	100.0	100.0	100.0
Delaware	HIGHMARK GRP	85.7	85.2	84.3	100.0	100.0	100.0
District of Columbia	CAREFIRST INC GRP	78.2	78.4	80.4	95.1	97.1	98.6
Florida	BLUE CROSS AND BLUE SHIELD OF FLORIDA, INC.	73.3	52.9	57.2	99.5	94.8	95.1
Georgia	WELLPOINT INC GRP	61.3	not the largest	not the largest	100.0	92.1	97.9
Georgia	HUMANA GRP	not the largest	43.4	60.3			
Illinois	HCSC GRP	68.7	88.4	95.0	100.0	100.0	100.0
Indiana	WELLPOINT INC GRP	91.6	99.3	100.0	100.0	100.0	100.0
Iowa	COOPORTUNITY HEALTH	70.5	not the largest	not the largest	100.0	100.0	100.0
Iowa	UNITEDHEALTH GRP	not the largest	70.0	not the largest			

Table 8. (Continued)

State	Name	Market share of the largest single issuer (%) (2015)	Market share of the largest single issuer (%) (2016)	Market share of the largest single issuer (%) (2017)	Market share of the largest three issuers (%) (2015)	Market share of the largest three issuers (%) (2016)	Market share of the largest three issuers (%) (2017)
Iowa	SANFORD HEALTH PLAN/SANFORD HEALTH PLAN OF MINNESOTA	not the largest	not the largest	46.7			
Kansas	BCBS OF KS GRP	98.3	99.0	94.7	100.0	100.0	100.0
Kentucky	KENTUCKY HEALTH COOPERATIVE	42.3	not the largest	not the largest	94.5	98.5	100.0
Kentucky	WELLPOINT INC GRP	not the largest	65.8	98.1			
Louisiana	LOUISIANA HLTH SERV GRP	80.4	95.2	91.5	100.0	100.0	100.0
Maine	MAINE COMMUNITY HEALTH OPTIONS	89.4	76.6	49.3	100.0	100.0	100.0
Maryland	UNITEDHEALTH GRP	40.7	37.2	43.8	76.3	82.3	92.1
Michigan	BCBS OF MI GRP	58.1	74.6	83.8	86.6	92.4	99.9
Minnesota	BCBS OF MN GRP	a	100.0	100.0	a	100.0	100.0
Mississippi	UNITEDHEALTH GRP	100.0	100.0	100.0	100.0	100.0	100.0
Missouri	WELLPOINT INC GRP	90.9	90.3	87.8	100.0	100.0	100.0
Montana	HCSC GRP	55.4	61.8	not the largest	100.0	100.0	100.0
Montana	PACIFICSOURCE HLTH PLAN GRP	not the largest	not the largest	59.6			
Nebraska	BLUE CROSS AND BLUE SHIELD OF NEBRASKA	79.6	100.0	100.0	100.0	100.0	100.0

State	Name	Market share of the largest single issuer (%) (2015)	Market share of the largest single issuer (%) (2016)	Market share of the largest single issuer (%) (2017)	Market share of the largest three issuers (%) (2015)	Market share of the largest three issuers (%) (2016)	Market share of the largest three issuers (%) (2017)
Nevada	NEVADA HEALTH CO-OP	100.0	not the largest	not the largest	100.0	100.0	100.0
Nevada	WELLPOINT INC GRP	not the largest	100.0	100.0			
New Hampshire	MAINE COMMUNITY HEALTH OPTIONS	60.0	55.5	not the largest	99.0	99.7	96.5
New Hampshire	WELLPOINT INC GRP	not the largest	not the largest	64.5			
New Jersey	BCBS OF NJ GRP	62.0	70.3	86.4	100.0	100.0	100.0
New Mexico	NEW MEXICO HEALTH CONNECTIONS	67.4	68.8	63.2	100.0	100.0	100.0
New York	FREELANCERS HEALTH SERVICE CORPORATION	33.0	not the largest	not the largest	73.0	61.8	66.2
New York	LIFETIME HLTHCARE GRP	not the largest	35.3	34.1			
North Carolina	BLUE CROSS AND BLUE SHIELD OF NORTH CAROLINA	100.0	100.0	100.0	100.0	100.0	100.0
North Dakota	NORIDIAN MUTUAL INSURANCE COMPANY	80.8	79.2	56.4	100.0	100.0	100.0
Ohio	MEDICAL MUTUAL OF OHIO	29.0	not the largest	not the largest	59.2	71.4	97.9
Ohio	WELLPOINT INC GRP	not the largest	46.7	82.7			
Oklahoma	HCSC GRP	84.5	81.5	76.6	100.0	100.0	100.0

Table 8. (Continued)

State	Name	Market share of the largest single issuer (%) (2015)	Market share of the largest single issuer (%) (2016)	Market share of the largest single issuer (%) (2017)	Market share of the largest three issuers (%) (2015)	Market share of the largest three issuers (%) (2016)	Market share of the largest three issuers (%) (2017)
Oregon	FREELANCERS CONSUMER OPERATED AND ORIENTED PROGRAM OF OREGON	70.9	not the largest	not the largest	92.5	83.2	93.7
Oregon	PACIFICSOURCE HLTH PLAN GRP	not the largest	32.5	not the largest			
Oregon	PROVIDENCE HEALTH PLAN	not the largest	not the largest	45.8			
Pennsylvania	HIGHMARK GRP	41.2	40.5	not the largest	88.7	79.6	87.1
Pennsylvania	INDEPENDENCE HEALTH GROUP, INC.	not the largest	not the largest	40.3			
Rhode Island	BLUE CROSS & BLUE SHIELD OF RHODE ISLAND	83.3	80.1	83.5	100.0	100.0	100.0
South Carolina	BCBS OF SC GRP	76.2	100.0	100.0	100.0	100.0	100.0
South Dakota	AVERA HEALTH PLANS, INC.	68.6	71.8	77.6	100.0	100.0	100.0
Tennessee	BCBS OF TN INC	50.9	100.0	100.0	100.0	100.0	100.0
Texas	HCSC GRP	97.0	95.1	99.2	100.0	100.0	100.0
Vermont	BCBS OF VT GRP	89.8	89.9	87.8	100.0	100.0	100.0
Virginia	WELLPOINT INC GRP	70.6	60.9	59.3	100.0	95.3	95.0
Washington	OREGON DENTAL GRP	72.9	not the largest	not the largest	100.0	100.0	100.0

State	Name	Market share of the largest single issuer (%) (2015)	Market share of the largest single issuer (%) (2016)	Market share of the largest single issuer (%) (2017)	Market share of the largest three issuers (%) (2015)	Market share of the largest three issuers (%) (2016)	Market share of the largest three issuers (%) (2017)
Washington	UNITEDHEALTH GRP	not the largest	49.5	68.9			
West Virginia	HIGHMARK GRP	100.0	100.0	100.0	100.0	100.0	100.0
Wisconsin	COMMON GROUND HEALTHCARE COOPERATIVE	28.6	not the largest	not the largest	53.5	55.3	61.0
Wisconsin	UNIVERSITY HEALTH CARE & GUNDERSEN LUTHERAN GROUP	not the largest	19.6	not the largest			
Wisconsin	WISCONSIN PHYSICIANS SERV INS GRP	not the largest	not the largest	21.8			
Wyoming	BLUE CROSS BLUE SHIELD OF WYOMING	88.7	100.0	100.0	100.0	100.0	100.0

Legend: — This symbol indicates that this issuer was not the largest in that year.

Source: GAO analysis of data from the Centers for Medicare & Medicaid Services and states. | GAO-19-306.

Note: This table excludes Hawaii, Idaho, Massachusetts, and Utah, as we did not have SHOP data for these states. Where multiple issuers in a state shared a parent company, we aggregated the individual issuers to the parent company level. We calculated issuers' market share using covered life-years, which measure the average number of lives insured, including dependents, during the reporting year. We measured market share in Oregon and Washington's SHOP exchange using covered lives, as these states were unable to provide covered life-years data. SHOP plans can begin at any time of year and generally continue for 12 months after the start date. Therefore, coverage can cross calendar years. We report SHOP enrollment by calendar year, which could, therefore, include enrollment with an issuer that had exited the SHOP market in a given year but is still providing coverage to enrollees whose plans began in the prior calendar year. We reprinted issuer names as they were reported in the data from the Centers for Medicare & Medicaid Services.

[a]Data were not available from Minnesota for 2015.

APPENDIX V: NUMBER AND MARKET SHARE OF LARGEST ISSUERS PARTICIPATING IN EACH STATE'S OVERALL INDIVIDUAL MARKET

The two tables below present information on the participation of issuers in each state's overall individual health insurance market from 2011 to 2016, and the market share of the largest and three largest issuers from 2014 to 2016.

Table 9. Number of Issuers in Each State's Overall Individual Health Insurance Market, 2011-2016

State	Number of issuers (2011)	Number of issuers (2012)	Number of issuers (2013)	Number of issuers (2014)	Number of issuers (2015)	Number of issuers (2016)
Alabama	27	22	23	17	16	11
Alaska	13	13	14	12	10	7
Arizona	30	26	24	27	23	17
Arkansas	32	26	24	21	19	16
California	45	34	30	33	31	27
Colorado	35	29	25	26	24	19
Connecticut	26	20	19	17	15	11
Delaware	20	17	16	14	13	10
District of Columbia	18	18	18	16	13	10
Florida	40	33	31	28	30	22
Georgia	38	32	31	29	25	18
Hawaii	14	15	12	10	9	7
Idaho	23	22	19	18	17	14
Illinois	42	37	34	30	25	21
Indiana	37	30	28	23	23	19
Iowa	33	27	25	21	19	14
Kansas	35	30	28	24	20	15
Kentucky	27	22	23	21	21	17
Louisiana	34	26	26	24	22	16

State	Number of issuers (2011)	Number of issuers (2012)	Number of issuers (2013)	Number of issuers (2014)	Number of issuers (2015)	Number of issuers (2016)
Maine	20	18	18	15	12	9
Maryland	27	24	23	19	18	15
Massachusetts	31	29	28	25	25	20
Michigan	41	33	33	31	29	22
Minnesota	36	29	26	25	25	18
Mississippi	30	25	22	21	18	14
Missouri	37	31	31	25	23	18
Montana	25	22	21	20	16	13
Nebraska	31	28	26	25	19	16
Nevada	24	20	21	19	19	15
New Hampshire	20	17	15	13	14	9
New Jersey	24	24	20	19	19	16
New Mexico	28	24	22	18	18	14
New York	38	32	28	32	33	27
North Carolina	31	26	25	22	18	15
North Dakota	21	20	19	13	12	10
Ohio	43	36	34	32	29	24
Oklahoma	30	26	25	23	21	16
Oregon	31	28	25	29	25	21
Pennsylvania	38	34	36	33	31	24
Rhode Island	14	12	13	11	9	7
South Carolina	31	24	22	20	17	15
South Dakota	30	26	25	17	14	11
Tennessee	33	29	26	23	20	15
Texas	50	40	36	38	37	32
Utah	24	19	19	19	17	14
Vermont	16	14	12	10	6	5
Virginia	32	29	29	29	26	21
Washington	30	27	25	24	23	19
West Virginia	27	25	24	19	18	15
Wisconsin	42	38	35	35	31	24
Wyoming	25	23	21	16	14	11

Source: GAO analysis of data from the Centers for Medicare & Medicaid Services. │GAO-19-306.

Note: Where multiple issuers in a state shared a parent company, we aggregated the individual issuers to the parent company level.

Table 10. Market Share of the Single Largest and Three Largest Issuers in Each State's Overall Individual Health Insurance Market, 2014-2016

State	Name	Market share of the largest single issuer (%) (2014)	Market share of the largest single issuer (%) (2015)	Market share of the largest single issuer (%) (2016)	Market share of the largest three issuers (%)	Market share of the largest three issuers (%)	Market share of the largest three issuers (%)
Alabama	BCBS OF AL GRP	90.3	85.7	76.4	98.1	99.3	99.6
Alaska	OREGON DENTAL GRP	not the largest	48.5	54.1	92.0	98.0	99.7
	PREMERA BLUE CROSS GROUP	54.2	not the largest	not the largest			
Arizona	BLUE CROSS AND BLUE SHIELD OF ARIZONA, INC.	41.5	42.2	42.0	82.9	74.8	80.1
Arkansas	ARKANSAS BCBS GRP	79.1	73.6	68.1	94.4	93.5	89.9
California	WELLPOINT INC GRP	35.0	30.9	30.3	82.4	82.3	85.3
Colorado	COLORADO HEALTH INSURANCE COOPERATIVE, INC.	not the largest	23.1	not the largest	56.0	63.5	79.9
	KAISER FOUNDATION GRP	not the largest	not the largest	35.6			
	WELLPOINT INC GRP	23.7	not the largest	not the largest			
Connecticut	HIP INS GRP	not the largest	45.1	53.6	86.2	86.6	92.2
	WELLPOINT INC GRP	36.5	not the largest	not the largest			
Delaware	HIGHMARK GRP	71.7	88.7	89.2	95.5	98.5	99.5
District of Columbia	CAREFIRST INC GRP	76.7	80.8	86.3	94.7	96.5	98.9

State	Name	Market share of the largest single issuer (%) (2014)	Market share of the largest single issuer (%) (2015)	Market share of the largest single issuer (%) (2016)	Market share of the largest three issuers (%)	Market share of the largest three issuers (%)	Market share of the largest three issuers (%)
Florida	BLUE CROSS AND BLUE SHIELD OF FLORIDA, INC.	40.4	33.6	43.6	75.3	65.9	69.3
Georgia	HUMANA GRP	46.9	46.3	31.5	84.6	83.5	72.3
Hawaii	HAWAII MEDICAL SERVICE ASSOCIATION	52.1	57.1	60.4	99.7	99.8	99.9
Idaho	BLUE CROSS OF IDAHO HEALTH SERVICE, INC.	59.7	60.0	49.4	92.1	89.1	86.0
Illinois	HCSC GRP	77.9	80.6	65.6	88.7	89.5	83.0
Indiana	WELLPOINT INC GRP	59.0	43.9	33.3	81.5	74.9	68.3
Iowa	WELLMARK GROUP	70.5	68.5	66.5	93.2	97.6	98.8
Kansas	AETNA GRP	38.1	not the largest	not the largest	89.3	93.7	89.7
	BCBS OF KS GRP	not the largest	41.9	56.0			
Kentucky	WELLPOINT INC GRP	51.2	52.5	76.3	95.9	94.3	92.0
Louisiana	LOUISIANA HLTH SERV GRP	72.4	64.6	60.8	87.9	86.1	91.0
Maine	MAINE COMMUNITY HEALTH OPTIONS	54.9	70.8	61.8	98.7	99.0	99.1
Maryland	CAREFIRST INC GRP	76.4	86.0	77.2	93.9	97.3	95.6
Massachusetts	BCBS OF MA GRP	30.4	not the largest	not the largest	73.5	72.3	72.9
	TUFTS HEALTH PLAN	not the largest	29.7	36.2			
Michigan	BCBS OF MI GRP	57.9	55.8	52.3	75.0	77.5	81.9

Table 10. (Continued)

State	Name	Market share of the largest single issuer (%) (2014)	Market share of the largest single issuer (%) (2015)	Market share of the largest single issuer (%) (2016)	Market share of the largest three issuers (%)	Market share of the largest three issuers (%)	Market share of the largest three issuers (%)
Minnesota	BCBS OF MN GRP	52.1	68.4	44.7	86.4	89.9	89.5
Mississippi	MISSISSIPPI INS GRP	49.8	44.1	43.5	86.0	85.1	84.8
Missouri	AETNA GRP	32.0	37.8	26.7	77.2	76.8	69.9
Montana	HCSC GRP	56.0	56.8	70.4	84.9	92.1	99.6
Nebraska	BLUE CROSS AND BLUE SHIELD OF NEBRASKA	57.8	49.1	48.5	87.8	91.6	95.6
Nevada	UNITEDHEALTH GRP	46.6	49.9	58.5	80.7	82.9	93.3
New Hampshire	WELLPOINT INC GRP	91.4	64.5	38.7	98.9	89.9	77.7
New Jersey	BCBS OF NJ GRP	55.9	56.3	59.9	95.4	90.7	87.0
New Mexico	HCSC GRP	57.3	43.5	not the largest	95.1	93.4	93.9
	PRESBYTERIAN HLTHCARE SERV GRP	not the largest	not the largest	35.5			
New York	AMERICAN INTL GRP	14.6	not the largest	14.4	42.6	42.6	41.8
	FREELANCERS HEALTH SERVICE CORPORATION	not the largest	19.1	not the largest			
North Carolina	BLUE CROSS AND BLUE SHIELD OF NORTH CAROLINA	84.3	75.3	60.3	96.5	98.0	99.1
North Dakota	NORIDIAN MUTUAL INSURANCE COMPANY	83.1	77.6	74.5	96.2	95.1	99.3

State	Name	Market share of the largest single issuer (%) (2014)	Market share of the largest single issuer (%) (2015)	Market share of the largest single issuer (%) (2016)	Market share of the largest three issuers (%)	Market share of the largest three issuers (%)	Market share of the largest three issuers (%)
Ohio	MEDICAL MUTUAL OF OHIO	38.1	36.8	35.0	76.5	66.7	69.2
Oklahoma	HCSC GRP	76.4	87.8	89.6	91.8	96.9	99.6
Oregon	OREGON DENTAL GRP	49.1	40.7	not the largest	73.1	69.7	79.2
	PROVIDENCE HEALTH PLAN	not the largest	not the largest	43.8			
Pennsylvania	HIGHMARK GRP	40.7	45.2	not the largest	81.0	76.8	68.2
	INDEPENDENCE HEALTH GROUP, INC.	not the largest	not the largest	29.0			
Rhode Island	BLUE CROSS & BLUE SHIELD OF RHODE ISLAND	94.0	58.5	60.7	99.2	99.5	99.6
South Carolina	BCBS OF SC GRP	48.7	51.3	90.2	83.1	90.3	99.3
South Dakota	WELLMARK GROUP	69.4	61.7	49.2	89.1	93.5	96.8
Tennessee	BCBS OF TN INC	61.6	63.2	58.6	88.6	86.8	86.3
Texas	HCSC GRP	67.6	64.6	44.6	87.5	84.5	63.4
Utah	IHC INC GRP	46.4	50.6	61.0	84.6	80.4	91.2
Vermont	BCBS OF VT GRP	87.5	89.5	87.9	99.9	100.0	100.0
Virginia	WELLPOINT INC GRP	59.5	52.7	45.8	77.4	73.4	69.8
Washington	PREMERA BLUE CROSS GROUP	50.0	48.1	42.4	85.2	78.6	77.0
West Virginia	HIGHMARK GRP	77.8	90.5	90.9	94.2	98.4	98.8

Table 10. (Continued)

State	Name	Market share of the largest single issuer (%) (2014)	Market share of the largest single issuer (%) (2015)	Market share of the largest single issuer (%) (2016)	Market share of the largest three issuers (%)	Market share of the largest three issuers (%)	Market share of the largest three issuers (%)
Wisconsin	MOLINA HEALTHCARE INC GRP	not the largest	not the largest	20.2	49.1	42.9	50.0
	WISCONSIN PHYSICIANS SERV INS GRP	20.3	15.0	not the largest			
Wyoming	BLUE CROSS BLUE SHIELD OF WYOMING	37.0	58.9	94.7	82.2	92.8	99.2

Legend: — This symbol indicates that this issuer was not the largest in that year.

Source: GAO analysis of data from the Centers for Medicare & Medicaid Services. | GAO-19-306.

Note: Where multiple issuers in a state shared a parent company, we aggregated the individual issuers to the parent company level. We calculated issuers' market share using covered life-years, which measure the average number of lives insured, including dependents, during the reporting year. We reprinted issuer names as they were reported in the data from the Centers for Medicare & Medicaid Services.

APPENDIX VI: MARKET SHARE FOR CONSUMER OPERATED AND ORIENTED PLANS THAT PARTICIPATED IN THE EXCHANGES

Table 11 provides market share for the 23 consumer operated and oriented plans (CO-OPs) participating in state individual market and Small Business Health Options Program exchanges for 2015 through 2017. CO-OPs are new consumer-governed, nonprofit issuers created under the Patient Protection and Affordable Care Act. Out of the 23 CO-OPs originally operating in 2014, all but four, operating in five states, had ceased operations by the end of 2017.

Table 11. Market Share for Consumer Operated and Oriented Plans (CO-OPs) That Participated in the Individual Market and Small Business Health Options Program (SHOP) Exchanges, 2015-2017

CO-OP	State where CO-OP participated in the exchange	Individual exchange market share (%) (2015)	Individual exchange market share (%) (2016)	Individual exchange market share (%) (2017)	SHOP exchange market share (%) (2015)	SHOP exchange market share (%) (2016)	SHOP exchange market share (%) (2017)
CO-OPs that continued to operate as of December 2018 MONTANA HEALTH COOPERATIVE	Idaho	18.3	15.7	13.9	a	a	a
CO-OPs that continued to operate as of December 2018 MAINE COMMUNITY HEALTH OPTIONS	Maine	81.0	67.5	42.4	89.4	76.6	49.3

Table 11. (Continued)

CO-OP	State where CO-OP participated in the exchange	Individual exchange market share (%) (2015)	Individual exchange market share (%) (2016)	Individual exchange market share (%) (2017)	SHOP exchange market share (%) (2015)	SHOP exchange market share (%) (2016)	SHOP exchange market share (%) (2017)
CO-OPs that continued to operate as of December 2018 MONTANA HEALTH COOPERATIVE	Montana	36.8	27.1	37.7	13.4	3.7	<0.1
CO-OPs that continued to operate as of December 2018 NEW MEXICO HEALTH CONNECTIONS	New Mexico	34.8	31.6	23.8	67.4	68.8	63.2
CO-OPs that continued to operate as of December 2018 COMMON GROUND HEALTHCARE COOPERATIVE	Wisconsin	17.1	6.7	12.1	28.6	18.1	13.3
CO-OPs that ceased to operate COMPASS COOPERATIVE HEALTH PLAN, INC.[b]	Arizona	28.5	*	*	10.0	<0.1	*
CO-OPs that ceased to operate COLORADO HEALTH INSURANCE COOPERATIVE, INC.	Colorado	43.0	*	*	15.7	*	*
CO-OPs that ceased to operate HEALTHYCT	Connecticut	15.8	10.9	*	34.0	44.0	0.6
CO-OPs that ceased to operate LAND OF LINCOLN MUTUAL HEALTH INSURANCE COMPANY	Illinois	11.4	7.2	*	28.9	4.4	*

CO-OP	State where CO-OP participated in the exchange	Individual exchange market share (%) (2015)	Individual exchange market share (%) (2016)	Individual exchange market share (%) (2017)	SHOP exchange market share (%) (2015)	SHOP exchange market share (%) (2016)	SHOP exchange market share (%) (2017)
CO-OPs that ceased to operate COOPORTUNITY HEALTH	Iowa	2.1	*	*	70.5	*	*
CO-OPs that ceased to operate KENTUCKY HEALTH CARE COOPERATIVE, INC.	Kentucky	64.3	*	*	42.3	1.5	*
CO-OPs that ceased to operate LOUISIANA HEALTH COOPERATIVE, INC.	Louisiana	14.0	*	*	10.3	*	*
CO-OPs that ceased to operate EVERGREEN HEALTH COOPERATIVE, INC.	Maryland	2.8	6.4	*	16.4	15.8	2.9
CO-OPs that ceased to operate MINUTEMAN HEALTH, INC.	Massachusetts	2.7	1.9	1.7	a	a	a
CO-OPs that ceased to operate CONSUMERS MUTUAL INSURANCE OF MICHIGAN	Michigan	1.8	*	*	4.4	*	*
CO-OPs that ceased to operate COOPORTUNITY HEALTH	Nebraska	4.6	*	*	20.4	*	*
CO-OPs that ceased to operate NEVADA HEALTH COOPERATIVE	Nevada	26.9	*	*	100.0	*	*
CO-OPs that ceased to operate MINUTEMAN HEALTH, INC.	New Hampshire	17.2	30.0	43.5	1.0	0.3	3.5

Table 11. (Continued)

CO-OP	State where CO-OP participated in the exchange	Individual exchange market share (%) (2015)	Individual exchange market share (%) (2016)	Individual exchange market share (%) (2017)	SHOP exchange market share (%) (2015)	SHOP exchange market share (%) (2016)	SHOP exchange market share (%) (2017)
CO-OPs that ceased to operate MAINE COMMUNITY HEALTH OPTIONS[c]	New Hampshire	6.7	4.0	*	60.0	55.5	3.8
CO-OPs that ceased to operate FREELANCERS COOP OF NEW JERSEY	New Jersey	20.6	7.2	*	*	2.6	*
CO-OPs that ceased to operate FREELANCERS HEALTH SERVICE CORPORATION	New York	17.7	*	*	33.1	*	*
CO-OPs that ceased to operate COORDINATED HEALTH MUTUAL, INC.	Ohio	5.8	2.5	*	15.7	9.0	*
CO-OPs that ceased to operate COMMUNITY CARE OF OREGON, INC.	Oregon	7.7	4.1	*	2.5	2.4	*
CO-OPs that ceased to operate FREELANCERS CONSUMER OPERATED AND ORIENTED PROGRAM OF OREGON, INC.	Oregon	2.5	*	*	70.9	*	*
CO-OPs that ceased to operate CONSUMERS' CHOICE HEALTH INSURANCE COMPANY	South Carolina	42.5	*	*	23.8	*	*

CO-OP	State where CO-OP participated in the exchange	Individual exchange market share (%) (2015)	Individual exchange market share (%) (2016)	Individual exchange market share (%) (2017)	SHOP exchange market share (%) (2015)	SHOP exchange market share (%) (2016)	SHOP exchange market share (%) (2017)
CO-OPs that ceased to operate COMMUNITY HEALTH ALLIANCE MUTUAL INSURANCE COMPANY	Tennessee	16.8	*	*	49.1	*	*
CO-OPs that ceased to operate ARCHES MUTUAL INSURANCE COMPANY	Utah	23.7	*	*	a	a	a

Legend: * = CO-OP did not have exchange enrollment in this year.

Source: GAO analysis of data from the Centers for Medicare & Medicaid Services and states. │GAO-19-306.

Note: We calculated issuers' market share using covered life-years, which measure the average number of lives insured, including dependents, during the reporting year. We measured market share in Oregon's SHOP exchange using covered lives, as the state was unable to provide covered life-years data. SHOP plans can begin at any time of year and generally continue for 12 months after the start date. Therefore, coverage can cross calendar years. We report SHOP enrollment by calendar year, which could, therefore, include enrollment with an issuer that had exited the SHOP market in a given year but is still providing coverage to enrollees whose plans began in the prior calendar year. We reprinted issuer names as they were reported in the data from the Centers for Medicare & Medicaid Services.

[a]This state did not provide us with SHOP data for this year.

[b]The CO-OP in Arizona also offered coverage under another name, Compass Cooperative Mutual Health Network, Inc., which had 1 percent market share in the individual exchange in 2015 before ceasing to operate.

[c]Community Health Options ceased to operate in New Hampshire beginning in 2017, but continued to operate in Maine.

APPENDIX VII: NUMBER AND MARKET SHARE OF LARGEST ISSUERS PARTICIPATING IN OVERALL SMALL GROUP HEALTH INSURANCE MARKET

The two tables below present information on the participation of issuers in each state's overall small group health insurance market from 2011 to 2016 and the market share of the largest and three largest issuers from 2014 to 2016.

Table 12. Number of Issuers in Each State's Overall Small Group Health Insurance Market, 2011-2016

State	Number of issuers (2011)	Number of issuers (2012)	Number of issuers (2013)	Number of issuers (2014)	Number of issuers (2015)	Number of issuers (2016)
Alabama	11	9	8	7	6	5
Alaska	7	6	6	6	5	4
Arizona	14	12	12	13	12	8
Arkansas	13	12	11	11	9	6
California	27	27	22	22	18	15
Colorado	11	11	9	9	10	8
Connecticut	11	8	7	9	9	7
Delaware	9	8	8	6	4	3
District of Columbia	9	7	6	6	7	5
Florida	16	13	14	13	12	9
Georgia	23	22	20	16	14	9
Hawaii	6	6	6	6	5	5
Idaho	11	10	11	10	11	10
Illinois	26	27	21	18	14	13
Indiana	27	26	24	20	18	16
Iowa	17	15	15	15	14	11
Kansas	17	14	13	10	8	6
Kentucky	10	8	9	8	8	5
Louisiana	12	10	11	10	8	6

State	Number of issuers (2011)	Number of issuers (2012)	Number of issuers (2013)	Number of issuers (2014)	Number of issuers (2015)	Number of issuers (2016)
Maine	8	6	5	5	6	5
Maryland	8	8	8	7	6	5
Massachusetts	13	14	13	13	11	12
Michigan	25	24	24	22	21	16
Minnesota	10	9	9	9	8	8
Mississippi	10	9	8	8	7	5
Missouri	19	19	17	13	11	8
Montana	10	9	8	9	8	6
Nebraska	17	15	12	12	8	7
Nevada	17	16	14	14	12	8
New Hampshire	9	7	6	7	6	6
New Jersey	7	7	6	7	7	7
New Mexico	11	8	7	7	4	4
New York	16	14	14	16	15	16
North Carolina	16	14	13	10	10	5
North Dakota	6	6	6	6	5	5
Ohio	30	29	25	24	22	17
Oklahoma	18	16	15	11	9	8
Oregon	9	8	8	13	14	14
Pennsylvania	21	19	19	16	14	11
Rhode Island	4	4	3	5	4	4
South Carolina	15	13	12	10	8	5
South Dakota	12	11	11	11	8	7
Tennessee	15	14	14	13	11	6
Texas	27	25	23	21	18	16
Utah	12	13	12	11	10	8
Vermont	4	3	3	3	3	3
Virginia	20	15	17	15	12	11
Washington	13	12	13	12	9	8
West Virginia	14	13	12	9	6	5
Wisconsin	27	26	24	24	23	21
Wyoming	9	7	7	7	6	4

Source: GAO analysis of data from the Centers for Medicare & Medicaid Services. │GAO-19-306.

Note: Where multiple issuers in a state shared a parent company, we aggregated the individual issuers to the parent company level.

Table 13. Market Share of the Single Largest and Three Largest Issuers in Each State's Overall Small Group Health Insurance Market, 2014-2016

State	Name	Market share of the largest single issuer (%) (2014)	Market share of the largest single issuer (%) (2015)	Market share of the largest single issuer (%) (2016)	Market share of the largest three issuers (%) (2014)	Market share of the largest three issuers (%) (2015)	Market share of the largest three issuers (%) (2016)
Alabama	BCBS OF AL GRP	97.3	97.0	96.8	99.9	99.9	100.0
Alaska	PREMERA BLUE CROSS GROUP	63.3	70.6	60.0	87.2	88.8	93.0
Arizona	BLUE CROSS AND BLUE SHIELD OF ARIZONA, INC.	22.8	25.0	not the largest	66.7	67.4	76.5
	UNITEDHEALTH GRP	not the largest	not the largest	30.7			
Arkansas	ARKANSAS BCBS GRP	65.7	66.8	61.0	97.8	97.9	98.0
California	KAISER FOUNDATION GRP	31.8	34.4	36.2	75.0	73.8	74.9
Colorado	WELLPOINT INC GRP	27.9	28.0	not the largest	78.9	77.3	81.6
	UNITEDHEALTH GRP	not the largest	not the largest	33.4			
Connecticut	WELLPOINT INC GRP	35.6	not the largest	not the largest	85.0	80.2	76.5
	HIP INS GRP	not the largest	37.5	33.4			
Delaware	HIGHMARK GRP	69.5	69.6	74.0	98.9	100.0	100.0

State	Name	Market share of the largest single issuer (%) (2014)	Market share of the largest single issuer (%) (2015)	Market share of the largest single issuer (%) (2016)	Market share of the largest three issuers (%) (2014)	Market share of the largest three issuers (%) (2015)	Market share of the largest three issuers (%) (2016)
District of Columbia	CAREFIRST INC GRP	81.7	82.9	82.0	96.2	96.6	96.6
Florida	BLUE CROSS AND BLUE SHIELD OF FLORIDA, INC.	36.0	35.2	37.0	84.0	81.7	83.1
Georgia	WELLPOINT INC GRP	29.9	29.0	not the largest	80.0	78.4	81.0
	HUMANA GRP	not the largest	not the largest	35.2			
Hawaii	HAWAII MEDICAL SERVICE ASSOCIATION	55.6	47.3	48.2	88.2	86.3	87.7
Idaho	BLUE CROSS OF IDAHO HEALTH SERVICE, INC.	49.9	53.7	47.7	89.8	95.6	97.7
Illinois	HCSC GRP	61.1	65.0	69.8	86.9	87.7	90.2
Indiana	WELLPOINT INC GRP	57.4	51.9	49.2	84.0	83.5	82.8
Iowa	WELLMARK GROUP	64.6	77.5	82.6	89.0	95.2	96.8
Kansas	BCBS OF KS GRP	61.9	63.8	63.7	82.5	84.0	85.8
Kentucky	WELLPOINT INC GRP	57.1	50.8	49.7	95.3	95.8	96.3
Louisiana	LOUISIANA HLTH SERV GRP	79.0	76.4	76.3	96.3	97.1	98.1
Maine	HARVARD PILGRIM HTH CARE GRP	41.2	43.8	37.3	98.4	93.4	83.3

Table 13. (Continued)

State	Name	Market share of the largest single issuer (%) (2014)	Market share of the largest single issuer (%) (2015)	Market share of the largest single issuer (%) (2016)	Market share of the largest three issuers (%) (2014)	Market share of the largest three issuers (%) (2015)	Market share of the largest three issuers (%) (2016)
Maryland	CAREFIRST INC GRP	68.9	67.3	67.5	96.4	90.8	92.4
Massachusetts	BCBS OF MA GRP	45.6	42.5	44.0	80.8	79.3	79.5
Michigan	BCBS OF MI GRP	55.6	52.4	55.2	79.5	78.9	83.0
Minnesota	BCBS OF MN GRP	36.5	not the largest	not the largest	88.7	92.0	92.0
	HEALTHPARTNERS GRP	not the largest	42.7	44.1			
Mississippi	MISSISSIPPI INS GRP	76.7	79.5	82.3	98.8	99.3	99.0
Missouri	WELLPOINT INC GRP	44.5	41.7	39.5	76.1	76.3	77.1
Montana	HCSC GRP	65.5	70.8	80.1	92.7	94.7	98.1
Nebraska	BLUE CROSS AND BLUE SHIELD OF NEBRASKA	42.5	38.2	50.0	80.4	89.3	95.0
Nevada	UNITEDHEALTH GRP	36.7	49.6	53.0	75.9	76.1	78.0
New Hampshire	WELLPOINT INC GRP	65.9	56.4	-	99.2	99.2	98.9
	HARVARD PILGRIM HTH CARE GRP	-	-	45.8			
New Jersey	BCBS OF NJ GRP	60.1	54.4	53.2	86.9	87.8	87.0
New Mexico	HCSC GRP	46.9	37.9	-	96.5	87.4	89.9
	PRESBYTERIAN HLTHCARE SERV GRP	-	-	31.8			

State	Name	Market share of the largest single issuer (%) (2014)	Market share of the largest single issuer (%) (2015)	Market share of the largest single issuer (%) (2016)	Market share of the largest three issuers (%) (2014)	Market share of the largest three issuers (%) (2015)	Market share of the largest three issuers (%) (2016)
New York	UNITEDHEALTH GRP	47.6	42.4	46.3	73.3	71.2	71.5
North Carolina	BLUE CROSS AND BLUE SHIELD OF NORTH CAROLINA	64.7	60.0	55.1	96.4	96.4	96.3
North Dakota	NORIDIAN MUTUAL INSURANCE COMPANY	84.4	82.6	83.5	98.4	99.4	99.7
Ohio	WELLPOINT INC GRP	38.8	37.3	36.2	80.6	80.1	80.9
Oklahoma	HCSC GRP	65.4	71.0	72.9	88.8	92.6	95.2
Oregon	PACIFICSOURCE HLTH PLAN GRP	18.6	-	-	50.4	45.4	56.6
	PROVIDENCE HEALTH PLAN	-	16.1	28.2			
Pennsylvania	INDEPENDENCE HEALTH GROUP, INC.	23.3	26.1	29.5	58.0	65.3	68.1
Rhode Island	BLUE CROSS & BLUE SHIELD OF RHODE ISLAND	78.0	78.8	82.4	100.0	99.6	99.0
South Carolina	BCBS OF SC GRP	75.8	80.3	85.8	97.2	97.5	98.4
South Dakota	WELLMARK GROUP	58.9	60.6	67.1	91.9	93.1	94.4
Tennessee	BCBS OF TN INC	69.2	65.4	63.4	96.2	97.1	98.4
Texas	HCSC GRP	57.0	60.0	56.9	87.5	89.7	91.4
Utah	IHC INC GRP	47.9	54.8	61.2	81.0	83.7	91.7
Vermont	BCBS OF VT GRP	82.2	88.7	89.2	100.0	100.0	100.0

Table 13. (Continued)

State	Name	Market share of the largest single issuer (%) (2014)	Market share of the largest single issuer (%) (2015)	Market share of the largest single issuer (%) (2016)	Market share of the largest three issuers (%) (2014)	Market share of the largest three issuers (%) (2015)	Market share of the largest three issuers (%) (2016)
Virginia	WELLPOINT INC GRP	44.1	44.6	43.9	73.3	72.8	70.2
Washington	PREMERA BLUE CROSS GROUP	45.2	56.3	53.2	77.6	81.7	86.0
West Virginia	HIGHMARK GRP	80.0	80.8	80.8	97.7	98.2	97.4
Wisconsin	UNITEDHEALTH GRP	32.6	33.6	39.4	55.7	56.2	56.6
Wyoming	BLUE CROSS BLUE SHIELD OF WYOMING	62.4	69.7	85.1	88.9	92.3	99.1

Legend: — This symbol indicates that this issuer was not the largest in that year.

Source: GAO analysis of data from the Centers for Medicare & Medicaid Services. | GAO-19-306.

Note: Where multiple issuers in a state shared a parent company, we aggregated the individual issuers to the parent company level. We calculated issuers' market share using covered life-years, which measure the average number of lives insured, including dependents, during the reporting year. We reprinted issuer names as they were reported in the data from the Centers for Medicare & Medicaid Services.

APPENDIX VIII: NUMBER AND MARKET SHARE OF LARGEST ISSUERS PARTICIPATING IN EACH STATE'S OVERALL LARGE GROUP HEALTH INSURANCE MARKET

The two tables below present information on the participation of issuers in each state's overall large group health insurance market from 2011 to 2016 and the market share of the single largest and three largest issuers from 2014 to 2016.

Table 14. Number of Issuers in Each State's Overall Large Group Health Insurance Market, 2011-2016

State	Number of issuers (2011)	Number of issuers (2012)	Number of issuers (2013)	Number of issuers (2014)	Number of issuers (2015)	Number of issuers (2016)
Alabama	7	8	7	7	7	8
Alaska	6	4	5	5	5	4
Arizona	13	13	12	12	12	11
Arkansas	10	10	9	10	10	7
California	32	28	24	25	24	23
Colorado	13	10	10	10	10	9
Connecticut	9	7	5	7	8	8
Delaware	6	6	6	5	4	5
District of Columbia	9	7	6	6	7	7
Florida	14	11	12	11	13	11
Georgia	16	16	16	14	15	13
Hawaii	7	7	7	7	6	6
Idaho	12	9	9	11	12	12
Illinois	20	21	18	18	19	18
Indiana	23	24	19	17	16	15
Iowa	14	14	14	12	13	13
Kansas	14	13	13	11	10	8
Kentucky	11	11	8	9	9	8
Louisiana	9	9	10	10	10	9
Maine	5	5	5	6	6	6
Maryland	9	7	6	6	7	6
Massachusetts	13	12	11	12	13	13
Michigan	24	25	24	25	25	19
Minnesota	14	11	11	9	11	11

Table 14. (Continued)

State	Number of issuers (2011)	Number of issuers (2012)	Number of issuers (2013)	Number of issuers (2014)	Number of issuers (2015)	Number of issuers (2016)
Mississippi	9	9	8	9	9	7
Missouri	18	16	15	14	14	11
Montana	8	6	7	8	7	8
Nebraska	10	8	9	10	10	7
Nevada	14	13	13	13	13	10
New Hampshire	6	6	6	6	5	8
New Jersey	9	10	8	9	8	8
New Mexico	10	8	7	6	6	6
New York	16	16	15	16	15	16
North Carolina	13	12	11	10	9	8
North Dakota	7	8	8	7	7	6
Ohio	20	21	18	21	21	20
Oklahoma	12	11	12	11	9	10
Oregon	12	12	11	11	15	13
Pennsylvania	17	17	18	17	16	15
Rhode Island	5	5	4	5	5	4
South Carolina	12	10	10	8	8	6
South Dakota	11	11	12	10	7	8
Tennessee	10	9	9	11	12	9
Texas	23	22	22	20	21	21
Utah	12	13	14	13	12	12
Vermont	4	3	4	4	3	3
Virginia	14	13	16	16	14	14
Washington	13	13	12	11	10	10
West Virginia	11	11	11	8	7	7
Wisconsin	28	27	27	26	25	23
Wyoming	6	6	7	7	7	6

Source: GAO analysis of data from the Centers for Medicare & Medicaid Services. | GAO-19-306.

Note: Where multiple issuers in a state shared a parent company, we aggregated the individual issuers to the parent company level.

Table 15. Market Share of the Single Largest Issuer and the Three Largest Issuers in Each State's Overall Large Group Health Insurance Market, 2014-2016

State	Name	Market share of the largest single issuer (%) (2014)	Market share of the largest single issuer (%) (2015)	Market share of the largest single issuer (%) (2016)	Market share of the largest three issuers (%) (2014)	Market share of the largest three issuers (%) (2015)	Market share of the largest three issuers (%) (2016)
Alabama	BCBS OF AL GRP	92.6	93.6	92.9	100.0	99.9	99.8
Alaska	PREMERA BLUE CROSS GROUP	85.5	84.2	83.9	99.6	97.8	98.5
Arizona	BLUE CROSS AND BLUE SHIELD OF ARIZONA, INC.	37.7	38.8	38.4	79.1	82.4	84.7
Arkansas	ARKANSAS BCBS GRP	79. 7	80.6	78.5	99.2	99.0	97.2
California	KAISER FOUNDATION GRP	44.3	45.7	47.9	74.0	74.3	73.6
Colorado	KAISER FOUNDATION GRP	46.8	46.1	48.5	85.0	84.8	85.0
Connecticut	WELLPOINT INC GRP	33.3	31.8	29.8	74.3	69.1	71.0
Delaware	HIGHMARK GRP	70.7	67.0	69.8	96.5	97.6	97.2
District of Columbia	AETNA GRP	39.8	39.6	37.4	82.2	82.6	81.3
Florida	BLUE CROSS AND BLUE SHIELD OF FLORIDA, INC.	54.3	53.2	49.4	86.5	87.5	87.8
Georgia	WELLPOINT INC GRP	43.7	46.0	44.1	78.4	80.8	78.3
Hawaii	HAWAII MEDICAL SERVICE ASSOCIATION	69.2	69.6	68.9	95.6	95.8	96.0
Idaho	BLUE CROSS OF IDAHO HEALTH SERVICE, INC.	68.6	68.1	65.5	96.0	95.1	93.9

Table 15. (Continued)

State	Name	Market share of the largest single issuer (%) (2014)	Market share of the largest single issuer (%) (2015)	Market share of the largest single issuer (%) (2016)	Market share of the largest three issuers (%) (2014)	Market share of the largest three issuers (%) (2015)	Market share of the largest three issuers (%) (2016)
Illinois	HCSC GRP	68.3	67.0	66.4	90.8	90.5	88.7
Indiana	WELLPOINT INC GRP	59.4	60.8	61.5	88.7	89.8	90.2
Iowa	WELLMARK GROUP	77.0	77.3	77.7	95.3	96.1	96.3
Kansas	BCBS OF KS GRP	54.4	57.1	51.6	88.7	89.0	91.2
Kentucky	WELLPOINT INC GRP	69.0	70.5	67.4	91.6	92.4	91.7
Louisiana	LOUISIANA HLTH SERV GRP	63.1	63.6	65.0	88.4	87.8	90.6
Maine	WELLPOINT INC GRP	71.9	70.0	70.3	95.1	95.6	96.2
Maryland	CAREFIRST INC GRP	67.9	66.3	65.5	90.5	90.3	91.1
Massachusetts	BCBS OF MA GRP	56.9	57.7	58.1	84.8	83.9	83.3
Michigan	BCBS OF MI GRP	52.7	54.3	54.9	77.9	78.2	80.0
Minnesota	HEALTHPARTNERS GRP	46.4	49.0	45. 8	94.8	95.0	96.0
Mississippi	MISSISSIPPI INS GRP	79.9	82.0	82.4	98.7	98.9	98.5
Missouri	WELLPOINT INC GRP	32.7	31.9	-	75.2	78.4	80.4
	BCBS OF KC GRP	-	-	29.2			
Montana	HCSC GRP	83.0	83.0	83.4	99.1	98.3	98.0
Nebraska	BLUE CROSS AND BLUE SHIELD OF NEBRASKA	78.2	79.1	77.1	97.5	98.9	99.3
Nevada	UNITEDHEALTH GRP	66.0	66.5	65.4	88.6	88.0	88.5

State	Name	Market share of the largest single issuer (%) (2014)	Market share of the largest single issuer (%) (2015)	Market share of the largest single issuer (%) (2016)	Market share of the largest three issuers (%) (2014)	Market share of the largest three issuers (%) (2015)	Market share of the largest three issuers (%) (2016)
New Hampshire	WELLPOINT INC GRP	55.6	57.5	57.0	98.0	99.3	98.2
New Jersey	BCBS OF NJ GRP	54.3	56.8	54.1	83.3	84.5	85.5
New Mexico	HCSC GRP	63.1	60.5	61. 8	99.6	98.4	95.1
New York	HIP INS GRP	26.9	-	-	55.2	47. 6	46.5
	LIFETIME HLTHCARE GRP	-	18.2	17.3			
North Carolina	BLUE CROSS AND BLUE SHIELD OF NORTH CAROLINA	74.6	72.2	68.7	96.3	96.1	96.3
North Dakota	NORIDIAN MUTUAL INSURANCE COMPANY	95.6	73.3	49.7	99.6	99.7	99.9
Ohio	WELLPOINT INC GRP	42.9	43.1	44.3	76.7	77.3	80.3
Oklahoma	HCSC GRP	54.3	54.0	52. 5	83.2	82.1	80.6
Oregon	KAISER FOUNDATION GRP	41.8	42.1	41.9	79.9	79.8	78.6
Pennsylvania	HIGHMARK GRP	34.2	35.9	35.1	72.0	72.4	68.0
Rhode Island	BLUE CROSS & BLUE SHIELD OF RHODE ISLAND	76.4	77.6	78.0	98.2	98.0	98.3
South Carolina	BCBS OF SC GRP	91.9	91.1	88.6	98.7	98.7	99.0
South Dakota	WELLMARK GROUP	58.8	58.3	55.1	90.0	89.5	85.7
Tennessee	BCBS OF TN INC	78.1	78.4	72.5	94.1	93.9	89.8
Texas	HCSC GRP	49.2	48.4	45.9	84.4	84.6	83.7
Utah	IHC INC GRP	43.1	43.1	42.1	86.2	84.6	81.9

<h1 style="text-align:center">Table 15. (Continued)</h1>

State	Name	Market share of the largest single issuer (%) (2014)	Market share of the largest single issuer (%) (2015)	Market share of the largest single issuer (%) (2016)	Market share of the largest three issuers (%) (2014)	Market share of the largest three issuers (%) (2015)	Market share of the largest three issuers (%) (2016)
Vermont	BCBS OF VT GRP	80.4	84.9	88.7	100.0	100.0	100.0
Virginia	WELLPOINT INC GRP	47.3	61.2	48.3	72.7	81.5	75.5
Washington	GROUP HLTH COOP GRP	31.0	32.1	32.6	86.2	84.8	85.3
West Virginia	HIGHMARK GRP	76.8	77.7	78.3	98.9	98.4	96.6
Wisconsin	DEAN HEALTH GRP	14.2	14.5	-	38.2	39.8	44.4
	WELLPOINT INC GRP	-	-	15.2			
Wyoming	BLUE CROSS BLUE SHIELD OF WYOMING	71.1	72.5	74.4	92.2	92.9	95.5

Legend: — This symbol indicates that this issuer was not the largest in that year.

Source: GAO analysis of data from the Centers for Medicare & Medicaid Services. │GAO-19-306.

Note: Where multiple issuers in a state shared a parent company, we aggregated the individual issuers to the parent company level. We calculated issuers' market share using covered life-years, which measure the average number of lives insured, including dependents, during the reporting year. We reprinted issuer names as they were reported in the data from the Centers for Medicare & Medicaid Services.

APPENDIX IX: ACCESSIBLE DATA

Data Tables

Accessible Data for Number of States Where the Three Largest Issuers Had at Least 80 Percent of Enrollment, by Market, 2011-2016

n/a	Large group market	Small group market	Individual market
Year	States where largest 3 issuers' share was at least 80 percent	States where largest 3 issuers' share was at least 80 percent	States where largest 3issuers' share was at least 80 percent
2011	40	36	33
2012	41	38	37
2013	40	37	39
2014	40	40	41
2015	43	38	37
2016	43	41	37

Accessible Data for Figure 1: Covered Life-Years Reported by Issuers to the Centers for Medicare & Medicaid Services in the Overall Individual, Small Group, and Large Group Health Insurance Markets, 2016

Category	Individual	Small group	Large group
Enrollment (in millions)	17,348,603	14,207,909	42,870,889

Accessible Data for Figure 2: Number of States Where the Market Share of the Three Largest Issuers Was at Least 80 Percent, Overall Individual Market, 2011-2016

Year	Number of states
2011	33
2012	37
2013	39
2014	41
2015	37
2016	37

Accessible Data for Figure 3: Percentage Point Change in Market Share Held by the Three Largest Issuers from 2014 to 2016, by State, Overall Individual Market

State	Percentage point change
Colorado[a]	23.9
Wyoming[a]	17.0
South Carolina[a]	16.2
Montana[a]	14.8
Nevada[a]	12.6
Alaska[a]	7.8
Nebraska[a]	7.8
Oklahoma[a]	7.8
South Dakota[a]	7.7
Michigan[a]	7.0
Utah[a]	6.6
Oregon	6.1
Connecticut[a]	5.9
Iowa[a]	5.6
West Virginia[a]	4.6
District of Columbia[a]	4.2
Delaware[a]	4.0
Louisiana[a]	3.1
Minnesota[a]	3.1
North Dakota[a]	3.1
California[a]	2.9
North Carolina[a]	2.6
Maryland[a]	1.7
Alabama[a]	1.5
Wisconsin	1.0
Kansas[a]	0.4
Maine[a]	0.4
Rhode Island[a]	0.4
Hawaii[a]	0.2
Vermont[a]	0.1
Massachusetts	-0.6
New York	-0.8
New Mexico[a]	-1.1
Mississippi[a]	-1.2
Tennessee[a]	-2.3
Arizona[a]	-2.8
Kentucky[a]	-3.9
Arkansas[a]	-4.5

State	Percentage point change
Illinois[a]	-5.7
Florida	-6.0
Idaho[a]	-6.1
Missouri	-7.3
Ohio	-7.3
Virginia	-7.6
Washington	-8.2
New Jersey[a]	-8.4
Georgia	-12.3
Pennsylvania	-12.8
Indiana	-13.3
New Hampshire	-21.2
Texas	-24.1

Accessible Data for Figure 4: Extent to Which the Three Largest Individual Market Exchange Issuers Had at Least 80 Percent Market Share, on Average, in 49 States' Rating Areas, 2015-2017

Group	Concentration category	Number of states (2015)	Number of states (2016)	Number of states (2017)
Not Highly Concentrated	On average, three largest issuers held less than 80% market share	2	3	2
Highly Concentrated	On average, three largest issuers held at least 80% market share	31	25	15
	On average, state had three or fewer issuers, thereby accounting for, on average, 100% or nearly 100% market share[a]	16	21	32

Accessible Data for Figure 5: Percentage Point Change in Average Market Share of the Largest Individual Market Exchange Issuer across Rating Areas from 2015 to 2017, by State

State	Percentage point change in market share
Arizona[a]	59.5
South Carolina[a]	40.8
Wyoming[a]	38.7
Mississippi[a]	33.5
Alaska[a]	28.7

(Continued)

State	Percentage point change in market share
New Mexico[a]	26.2
North Carolina[a]	26.0
Kansas[a]	24.6
Nevada[a]	19.3
Alabama[a]	19.1
Connecticut[a]	17.9
Louisiana[a]	16.4
South Dakota[a]	14.8
New Jersey[a]	14.3
Nebraska[a]	13.3
Oregon[a]	13.1
Florida[a]	11.8
New York	10.6
Missouri[a]	7.3
Utah[a]	7.1
Colorado[a]	6.6
Pennsylvania[a]	6.3
Tennessee[a]	6.1
Wisconsin[a]	5.7
Virginia[a]	5.4
Massachusetts	5.1
Montana[a]	4.9
Rhode Island[a]	4.4
Ohio	4.0
Oklahoma[a]	2.5
District of Columbia[a]	2.2
Kentucky[a]	2.1
North Dakota[a]	-1.1
California	-1.4
Indiana	-1.4
Georgia[a]	-2.2
Idaho[a]	-4.7
Illinois[a]	-7.6
Vermont[a]	-11.0
Michigan[a]	-11.7
Maryland[a]	-12.0
Texas[a]	-16.0
Washington	-16.3
New Hampshire	-16.7
West Virginia[a]	-18.9

State	Percentage point change in market share
Iowa[a]	-24.8
Arkansas[a]	-25.5
Delaware[a]	-37.2
Maine	-38.6

Accessible Data for Figure 6: Number of States Where the Market Share of the Three Largest Issuers Was at Least 80 Percent, Overall Small Group Market, 2011- 2016

Year	Number of states
2011	36
2012	38
2013	37
2014	40
2015	38
2016	41

Accessible Data for Figure 7: Percentage Point Change in Market Share Held by the Three Largest Issuers from 2014 to 2016, by State, Small Group Market

State	Percentage point change
Nebraska[a]	14.6
Utaha	10.7
Wyoming[a]	10.2
Pennsylvania	10.1
Arizona	9.8
Washington[a]	8.4
Idaho[a]	7.9
Iowa[a]	7.8
Oklahoma[a]	6.4
Oregon	6.2
Alaska[a]	5.8
Montana[a]	5.4
Texas[a]	3.9
Michigan[a]	3.5
Illinois[a]	3.3

(Continued)

State	Percentage point change
Kansas[a]	3.3
Minnesota[a]	3.3
Colorado[a]	2.7
South Dakota[a]	2.5
Tennessee[a]	2.2
Nevada	2.1
Louisiana[a]	1.8
North Dakota[a]	1.3
South Carolina[a]	1.2
Delaware[a]	1.1
Georgia[a]	1.0
Kentucky[a]	1.0
Missouri	1.0
Wisconsin	0.9
District of Columbia[a]	0.4
Ohio[a]	0.3
Arkansas[a]	0.2
Mississippi[a]	0.2
Alabama[a]	0.1
New Jersey[a]	0.1
Vermonta,[b]	0.0
California	-0.1
North Carolina[a]	-0.1
New Hampshire[a]	-0.3
West Virginia[a]	-0.3
Hawaii[a]	-0.5
Florida[a]	-0.9
Rhode Island[a]	-0.9
Indiana[a]	-1.2
Massachusetts[a]	-1.3
New York	-1.8
Virginia	-3.1
Maryland[a]	-4.0
New Mexico[a]	-6.6
Connecticut	-8.5
Maine[a]	-15.1

Accessible Data for Figure 8: Extent to Which the Three Largest Issuers Had at Least 80 Percent Market Share in 46 Small Business Health Options Program Exchanges, 2015-2017

Group	Concentration Category	Number of States (2015)	Number of States (2016)	Number of States (2017)
Not Highly Concentrated	Three largest issuers held less than 80% market share	4	3	2
Highly Concentrated	Three largest issuers held at least 80% market share	10	13	12
	State had three or fewer issuers, thereby accounting for 100% market share	32	30	32

Accessible Data for Figure 9: Percentage Point Change in Market Share of the Largest Small Group Exchange Issuer from 2015 to 2017 across 46 States

State	Percentage point change in market share
Kentucky[a]	55.8
Ohio[a]	53.7
Tennessee[a]	49.1
Connecticut[a]	44.5
Illinois[a]	26.3
Michigan[a]	25.7
New Jersey[a]	24.4
South Carolina[a]	23.8
Arizona[a]	23.1
Nebraska[a]	20.4
Wyoming[a]	11.3
Louisiana[a]	11.1
California[a]	10.3
South Dakota[a]	9
Indiana[a]	8.4
New Hampshire[a]	4.6
Montana[a]	4.1
Colorado[a]	3.4
Maryland	3
District of Columbia[a]	2.3
Texas[a]	2.2
New York	1.1

(Continued)

State	Percentage point change in market share
Rhode Island[a]	0.2
Alabamaa,[b]	0
Arkansasa,[b]	0
Mississippia,[b]	0
Nevadaa,[b]	0
North Carolinaa,[b]	0
West Virginiaa,[b]	0
Pennsylvania	-0.9
Georgia[a]	-1
Delaware[a]	-1.5
Vermont[a]	-2
Missouri[a]	-3.2
Kansas[a]	-3.6
Washington[a]	-4
New Mexico[a]	-4.2
Wisconsin	-6.8
Oklahoma[a]	-7.9
Virginia[a]	-11.3
Florida[a]	-16.2
Iowa	-23.8
North Dakota[a]	-24.4
Oregon	-25.1
Alaska[a]	-36.5
Maine	-40.1

Accessible Data for Figure 10: Number of States in Which the Three Largest Issuers Held at Least 80 Percent Market Share, Overall Large Group Market, 2011-2016

Year	Number of states
2011	40
2012	41
2013	40
2014	40
2015	43
2016	43

Accessible Data for Figure 11: Percentage Point Change in Market Share Held by the Three Largest Issuers from 2014 to 2016, by State, Large Group Market

State	Percentage point change in market share
Wisconsin	6.2
Arizona[a]	5.6
Missouri[a]	5.2
Ohio[a]	3.6
Wyoming[a]	3.3
Virgini[a]	2.8
Kansas[a]	2.5
New Jersey[a]	2.2
Louisiana[a]	2.2
Michigan[a]	2.1
Nebraska[a]	1.8
Indiana[a]	1.4
Florida[a]	1.3
Minnesota[a]	1.2
Iowa[a]	1.0
Maine[a]	1.0
Delaware[a]	0.7
Maryland[a]	0.6
Hawaii[a]	0.4
North Dakota[a]	0.3
South Carolina[a]	0.3
New Hampshire[a]	0.2
Kentucky[a]	0.1
Rhode Island[a]	0.1
Coloradoa,[b]	0.0
North Carolinaa,[b]	0.0
Vermonta,[b]	0.0
Georgia	-0.1
Nevada[a]	-0.1
Alabama[a]	-0.2
Mississippi[a]	-0.2
Californi[a]	-0.5
Texas[a]	-0.8
District of Columbia[a]	-0.9
Washington[a]	-0.9
Alaska[a]	-1.1
Montana[a]	-1.1

(Continued)

State	Percentage point change in market share
Oregon	-1.3
Massachusetts[a]	-1.5
Arkansas[a]	-2.0
Illinois[a]	-2.0
Idaho[a]	-2.1
West Virginia[a]	-2.3
Oklahoma[a]	-2.5
Connecticut	-3.3
Pennsylvani[a]	-4.0
South Dakota[a]	-4.3
Tennessee[a]	-4.3
Utah[a]	-4.3
New Mexico[a]	-4.5
New York	-8.6

INDEX

A

access, 49, 53, 56, 60, 61, 126, 129, 130, 132, 134, 139

accounting, ix, 8, 39, 64, 207, 211

active duty service obligations, viii, 30, 33

agencies, 48, 49, 50, 51, 52, 53, 54, 55, 58, 59, 61, 68, 69, 70, 71, 72, 73, 89, 91, 92, 94, 98, 99, 100, 102, 103, 104, 105, 112

air ambulance providers, vii, 2, 3, 4, 5, 6, 8, 9, 10, 11, 13, 14, 15, 16, 17, 19, 20, 21, 22, 23, 24, 25, 26

air ambulance services, vii, 2, 5, 6, 17, 18, 20, 22, 23, 25

air ambulance transports, vii, 2, 3, 5, 6, 7, 9, 10, 11, 17, 18, 19, 22, 23, 25

air ambulances, vii, 2, 4, 6, 10, 12

airports, 8, 9, 14, 15, 16

Alaska, 147, 151, 152, 156, 158, 160, 162, 169, 171, 173, 175, 180, 182, 192, 194, 199, 201

B

beneficiaries, viii, 30, 33, 34, 67, 74, 86, 87, 93

benefits, 23, 104, 132, 133

business processes, 34

C

Centers for Disease Control and Prevention, viii, 47, 50

challenges, 6, 22, 41, 61, 93, 96, 132

coding, 76, 77, 85, 88, 112

communication, 31, 37, 100

competition, ix, 124, 127, 133

compliance, 66, 67, 72, 73, 74, 88, 95, 96, 103, 105, 112

composition, 13, 38

Congress, viii, 13, 23, 30, 31, 33, 34, 35, 36, 38, 40, 41, 51, 54, 57, 127

Consolidated Appropriations Act, vii, 2, 5, 53

consumer protection, 25

consumers, ix, 5, 25, 124, 126, 133

cost, 2, 9, 10, 22, 23, 50, 57, 98, 134

criminal activity, 57
criminal investigations, 53
critically ill patients, vii, 2, 4

D

data collection, 58, 129, 172
data processing, 71
data set, vii, x, 2, 3, 7, 18, 19, 124
database, 7, 18
Department of Defense, 29, 31, 32, 33, 37
Department of Health and Human Services, viii, 2, 26, 49, 50, 53, 63, 67, 95, 107, 123, 126, 127
Department of Justice, 59
Department of Transportation (DOT), viii, 1, 2, 4, 6, 12, 13, 24, 25, 26
District of Columbia, 7, 53, 97, 127, 136, 137, 140, 143, 145, 147, 148, 150, 152, 153, 156, 157, 158, 160, 163, 169, 171, 172, 173, 175, 180, 182, 192, 195, 199, 201, 206, 208, 210, 211, 213
drug addict, 48, 55
drug addiction, 48, 55
drug control activities, 55
Drug Enforcement Administration, 50, 60
drug misuse, viii, 47, 48, 50
drug overdoses, viii, 47, 50
drug policy, v, viii, 47
drug treatment, 53
drugs, 48, 50, 51, 53, 54, 55, 56, 59

E

education, 22, 25, 29, 30, 33, 71, 93, 94, 99
emergency, vii, 2, 3, 4, 11, 19, 22, 24, 25, 35, 50, 57
emergency services, vii, 2, 3, 4, 19
employees, 24, 126, 134, 154
employers, 124, 126, 127, 132, 133, 134, 151, 154

end-stage renal disease, 9, 66
enrollment, ix, x, 64, 70, 71, 124, 126, 127, 128, 129, 130, 131, 133, 138, 144, 147, 151, 157, 161, 170, 172, 179, 191
equipment, 12, 63, 69, 87, 91, 112
evidence, 8, 34, 41, 52, 56, 61, 69, 72, 82, 100, 132
evidence-based policy, 61
executive branch, 58, 72
expenditures, 66, 70, 72

F

federal government, ix, 11, 50, 51, 61, 64, 72, 134
federal law, 3, 6, 12, 50, 154
financial, 2, 5, 19, 21, 23, 92, 93, 99
first responders, 11, 26
fiscal year, ix, 35, 51, 53, 57, 64, 66, 67, 68, 69, 70, 71, 73, 76, 82, 83, 84, 86, 88, 95, 97, 100, 111, 134
flexibility, ix, 64, 72
fraud, 51, 69, 71, 74, 81, 82, 92, 94, 100, 101, 102, 103, 104, 105

G

Georgia, 138, 156, 158, 160, 163, 169, 171, 173, 175, 180, 183, 192, 195, 199, 201, 207, 213
grant programs, 60
guidance, 67, 70, 72, 99

H

Hawaii, 129, 130, 139, 140, 143, 148, 150, 156, 158, 159, 160, 161, 163, 168, 169, 170, 172, 174, 179, 180, 183, 192, 195, 199, 201 health, vii, viii, ix, 2, 5, 6, 7, 9, 10, 11, 12, 19, 20, 22, 23, 24, 25, 30, 33, 34, 35, 50, 57, 60, 66, 67, 69, 72, 74, 80, 85, 86, 87, 88, 89, 91, 92, 94, 112, 113, 124, 125, 126, 127, 128, 131, 132, 133, 135, 139, 144, 151, 158, 173, 180, 192, 199

Health and Human Services, 4, 26, 53, 106

health care, v, vii, viii, 5, 9, 10, 11, 19, 20, 22, 25, 27, 29, 30, 33, 34, 35, 39, 40, 41, 57, 66, 67, 72, 106, 126, 127, 132, 133, 142, 151, 154

health care programs, 72

health care system, viii, 30

health insurance, vii, ix, 2, 5, 7, 9, 12, 20, 24, 66, 124, 125, 126, 127, 128, 132, 133, 135, 144, 151, 158, 173, 180, 192, 199

health insurance exchanges, ix, 124, 125, 126, 133, 135, 169

health insurance market, ix, 124, 126, 127, 132, 133, 134, 135, 144, 151, 180, 182, 192, 194, 199, 201, 205

health insurers, vii, 2, 6, 12, 23, 25

health risks, 134

health services, 74, 80, 87, 94, 113

health status, 134

hospice, 69, 85, 86, 87, 88

House of Representatives, 1, 4, 33, 47, 106, 107, 155, 156

Housing and Urban Development, 53

humanitarian missions, viii, 30, 33

I

illicit drug use, 48, 50, 54, 55, 56

improper payments, v, ix, 63, 64, 65, 66, 67, 68, 69, 70, 71, 72, 73, 75, 76, 77, 78, 79, 80, 81, 83, 85, 89, 92, 93, 94, 95, 96, 97, 98, 99, 100, 101, 102, 103, 104, 105, 111, 112

individuals, ix, 9, 20, 24, 39, 50, 61, 66, 124, 126, 127, 129, 134, 157

insurance plans, ix, 11, 12, 24, 124, 127

integrity, 65, 66, 68, 69, 74, 82, 86, 94, 95, 99

Iowa, 156, 159, 160, 163, 169, 171, 173, 175, 176, 180, 183, 189, 192, 195, 199, 202, 212

L

laboratory tests, 91

law enforcement, 51, 52, 54, 59, 100, 101

Louisiana, 144, 156, 159, 160, 164, 169, 171, 173, 176, 180, 183, 189, 192, 195, 199, 202

M

majority, 71, 76, 131, 132

management, 35, 61, 70, 91, 99

market concentration, ix, 124, 133

market share, x, 124, 125, 127, 128, 129, 130, 131, 135, 136, 137, 138, 139, 140, 141, 142, 143, 144, 145, 146, 147, 148, 149, 150, 151, 152, 153, 154, 158, 168, 169, 170, 172, 173, 179, 180, 186, 187, 188, 189, 190, 191, 192, 198, 199, 204, 207, 208, 209, 211, 212, 213, 214

marketplace, ix, 124

Maryland, vii, 2, 6, 20, 22, 26, 134, 157, 159, 160, 164, 169, 172, 173, 176, 181, 183, 189, 193, 196, 199, 202, 211

median, 3, 4, 19, 20, 138, 141, 142, 145, 149, 151

Medicaid, v, viii, ix, x, 2, 6, 9, 50, 63, 64, 65, 66, 67, 68, 69, 70, 71, 72, 73, 74, 75, 76, 77, 78, 79, 80, 81, 82, 84, 85, 86, 87, 88, 89, 90, 91, 92, 94, 95, 96, 97, 98, 99, 100, 101, 102, 103, 104, 105, 111, 112, 120, 123, 124, 125, 127, 133, 136, 137,

140, 143, 145, 146, 148, 150, 152, 153,
157, 159, 161, 168, 170, 172, 174, 179,
181, 186, 191, 193, 198, 200, 204, 205
medical, viii, ix, 6, 7, 12, 17, 21, 25, 29, 30,
31, 32, 33, 34, 35, 36, 37, 38, 39, 63, 64,
65, 66, 67, 68, 69, 70, 73, 74, 75, 76, 77,
78, 80, 82, 83, 85, 86, 87, 88, 91, 92, 93,
94, 96, 97, 98, 99, 100, 101, 103, 104,
105, 112, 127
medical care, 39
medical force readiness, viii, 30, 31, 32, 33,
35, 37, 38
medical personnel, viii, 30, 33, 36, 39
medical training, viii, 30, 33
Medicare, v, viii, ix, x, 2, 6, 9, 63, 64, 65,
66, 67, 68, 69, 71, 72, 73, 74, 75, 76, 77,
78, 79, 80, 81, 84, 85, 86, 87, 88, 89, 91,
92, 93, 94, 95, 97, 100, 102, 103, 104,
111, 112, 113, 118, 119, 123, 124, 125,
127, 133, 136, 137, 140, 143, 145, 146,
148, 150,152, 153, 157, 159, 161, 168,
170, 172, 174, 179, 181, 186, 191, 193,
198, 200, 204, 205
medication, 49, 50, 56, 60
mentally fit, viii, 30, 33
Mexico, vii, 2, 6, 21, 22, 25, 157, 159, 161,
165, 170, 172, 174, 177, 181, 184, 188,
193, 196, 200, 203
military, viii, 9, 29, 30, 31, 32, 33, 34, 35,
36, 37, 38, 39, 40
military physicians, viii, 30, 33
military servicemembers, viii, 30, 33
Missouri, 154, 157, 159, 160, 165, 169, 171,
174, 176, 181, 184, 193, 196, 200, 202,
207, 210
misuse, viii, 47, 48, 50, 51, 53, 60
Montana, vii, 2, 6, 21, 22, 23, 24, 152, 157,
159, 160, 165, 169, 171, 174, 176, 181,
184, 188, 193, 196, 200, 202
morphine, 50
multiple factors, 39, 135

N

National Defense Authorization Act, 29, 30,
32, 33, 37
national drug control, 51, 53, 57
National Drug Control Strategy, v, viii, ix,
47, 48, 49, 51, 52, 54, 55, 56, 57, 58, 62

O

Office of Management and Budget, 58, 64,
67, 70, 72
Office of National Drug Control Policy, 48,
50, 52
Office of the Inspector General, 63, 71
officials, vii, viii, ix, 2, 6, 7, 8, 21, 23, 24,
25, 26, 30, 32, 34, 35, 36, 37, 38, 39, 40,
41, 48, 52, 54, 58, 64, 68, 69, 70, 77, 82,
84, 87, 92, 93, 94, 95, 96, 97, 98, 99,
101, 102, 104, 128, 129, 131, 157, 172
out-of-network providers, vii, 2, 5
outpatient, 69, 71
outreach, 69, 80, 82, 94, 100
overdoses, viii, 47, 50, 51
oversight, viii, 13, 25, 30, 31, 32, 33, 34, 36,
37, 38, 40, 41, 68, 70

P

performance measurement, 57
physicians, viii, 11, 19, 24, 25, 30, 33, 35,
40, 70, 80, 82, 86, 92, 93, 113, 119
policy, viii, 12, 35, 38, 47, 51, 53, 54, 58,
74, 77, 86, 87, 88, 100, 102, 134
policymakers, 5
population, 7, 8, 17, 23, 131
PPACA, ix, 123, 124, 125, 126, 127, 133,
134
prevention, 48, 51, 52, 55
private health insurance data, vii, 2

private sector, 55
privately-insured patients, v, vii, 1, 2, 3, 5, 7, 9, 10, 18
providers, ix, 2, 3, 5, 6, 7, 9, 10, 11, 13, 14, 15, 16, 17, 19, 21, 22, 23, 24, 25, 26, 35, 50, 61, 64, 67, 69, 71, 72, 73, 74, 76, 78, 79, 82, 84, 86, 93, 94, 95, 98, 100, 101, 102, 103, 104, 105, 112, 132
public awareness, 26
public health, 50, 54, 59
public safety, 59

R

recommendations, ix, 13, 24, 25, 31, 32, 37, 38, 48, 49, 51, 52, 64, 76, 103, 105
requirements, viii, ix, 12, 13, 22, 30, 31, 32, 33, 34, 35, 36, 37, 38, 39, 40, 41, 48, 54, 56, 57, 59, 64, 65, 67, 68, 69, 70, 71, 73, 74, 77, 78, 86, 87, 88, 91, 92, 93, 94, 95, 96, 102, 103, 104
resources, 17, 49, 61, 98, 99, 105
response, 8, 50, 51, 59, 76, 79, 101, 127
risk, 2, 5, 23, 51, 66, 73, 89, 92, 93, 99, 101, 134
risks, 19, 40, 41, 65, 66, 68, 94, 98, 99, 102, 103, 105

S

servicemembers, viii, 30, 33, 36, 37
services, vii, 2, 3, 4, 5, 6, 7, 10, 11, 12, 17, 18, 19, 20, 22, 23, 25, 31, 33, 34, 35, 36, 37, 38, 39, 40, 60, 65, 67, 69, 72, 73, 74, 76, 80, 81, 84, 85, 86, 87, 88, 89, 92, 93, 94, 96, 98, 99, 102, 111, 112
South Dakota, 157, 159, 161, 167, 170, 172, 174, 178, 181, 185, 193, 197, 200, 203, 206, 208, 210, 211, 214
specific knowledge, 56
spending, ix, 64, 67, 98, 111

stakeholders, 11, 17, 22, 25, 26, 87, 95
statutory provisions, 52
strategic management, 40
substance use disorders, 51, 56

T

technical assistance, 99
technical comments, viii, 2, 26, 41, 104, 126, 154
training, viii, 30, 31, 32, 33, 34, 36, 37, 38, 39, 71
transport, 3, 4, 5, 11, 17, 19, 20, 23
transportation, 12
transports, vii, 2, 3, 4, 7, 8, 9, 10, 11, 13, 14, 16, 17, 18, 19, 20, 24, 25
treatment, 29, 32, 33, 34, 37, 48, 49, 51, 52, 55, 56, 60

U

United States, v, viii, 1, 4, 16, 29, 32, 47, 53, 55, 56, 57, 59, 63, 106, 123, 132, 151, 155

W

wartime, viii, 30, 33, 34, 35
Washington, 4, 12, 13, 17, 33, 39, 40, 50, 51, 52, 59, 67, 70, 72, 77, 84, 92, 94, 95, 99, 126, 130, 132, 134, 135, 138, 146, 148, 150, 151, 157, 159, 161, 167, 170, 172, 174, 178, 179, 181, 185, 193, 198, 200, 204, 207, 208
Wisconsin, 139, 151, 154, 157, 159, 161, 167, 168, 170, 172, 174, 179, 181, 186, 188, 193, 198, 200, 204, 206, 210, 212, 213
workers, 13, 23, 151

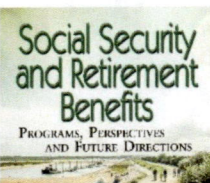